Introduction to
Brain-Compatible
Learning

Second Edition

To you who are just getting started, may you enjoy
both the journey and the results.
Many thanks to my wife, Diane, for her priceless support.

"If the brain were so simple we could understand it,
we would be so simple, we couldn't."

—Lyall Watson

Introduction to
Brain-Compatible
Learning

Second Edition

Eric Jensen

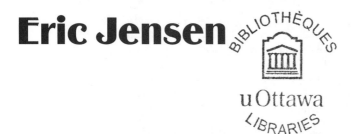

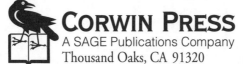

CORWIN PRESS
A SAGE Publications Company
Thousand Oaks, CA 91320

Copyright © 2007 by Corwin Press

For information:

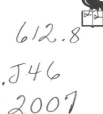

Corwin Press
A SAGE Publications Company
2455 Teller Road
Thousand Oaks, California 91320
www.corwinpress.com

SAGE Publications Ltd.
1 Oliver's Yard
55 City Road
London, EC1Y 1SP
United Kingdom

SAGE Publications India Pvt. Ltd.
B 1/I 1 Mohan Cooperative
    Industrial Area
Mathura Road, New Delhi 110 044
India

SAGE Publications Asia-Pacific Pte. Ltd.
33 Pekin Street #02-01
Far East Square
Singapore 048763

Printed in the United States of America.

Library of Congress Cataloging-in-Publication Data

Jensen, Eric, 1950-
Introduction to brain-compatible learning / Eric Jensen.—2nd ed.
    p. cm.
Includes bibliographical references and index.
ISBN 978-1-4129-5407-5 (cloth: alk. paper)
ISBN 978-1-4129-5418-1 (pbk. : alk. paper)
    1. Learning—Physiological aspects—Popular works. 2. Brain—Popular works.
I. Title.
QP408.J46 2007
12.8—dc22

                          2006102763

This book is printed on acid-free paper.

07 08 09 10 11 10 9 8 7 6 5 4 3 2 1

Acquisitions Editor:	Rachel Livsey
Editorial Assistant:	Phyllis Cappello
Production Editor:	Jenn Reese
Copy Editor:	Barbara Coster
Typesetter:	C&M Digitals (P) Ltd.
Proofreader:	Joyce Li
Indexer:	Ellen Slavitz
Cover Designer:	Lisa Miller

CONTENTS

Part II: The Foundation for Teaching Is Principles, Not Strategies

Part III: So What; Now What?

ACKNOWLEDGMENTS

The contributions of the following reviewers are gratefully acknowledged:

Marilee Sprenger
Educational Neuroscience
　Consultant
Brainlady
Peoria, IL

Steve Hutton
Area Coordinator for the Kentucky
　Center for Instructional Discipline
Villa Hills, KY

Susan Stone Kessler
Assistant Principal
Hillsboro High School
Metropolitan Nashville
　Public Schools
Nashville, TN

Andrea F. Rosenblatt
Associate Professor
Graduate Reading Program
Barry University
Miami Shores, FL

Beverly Ginther
Staff Development Coordinator
Minnetonka Public Schools
Minnetonka, MN

David A. Sousa
Educational Consultant
Palm Beach, FL

Mike Greenwood
District Teacher Leader
Windsor Public Schools
Windsor, CT

ABOUT THE AUTHOR

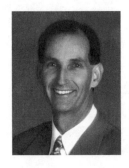 **Eric Jensen** is a staff developer and former teacher who has taught at all levels of education—from elementary through university. In 1981, he cofounded SuperCamp, the United States' first and largest brain-compatible learning program, now with over 45,000 graduates. He's authored *Brain-Based Learning, Brain-Compatible Strategies, Teaching With the Brain in Mind, Enriching the Brain,* and *SuperTeaching.* He is currently a member of the Society for Neuroscience and the New York Academy of Sciences and is completing his PhD in psychology. He speaks at conferences and offers in-depth trainings at www.jensenlearning.com. He remains deeply committed to making a positive, significant, lasting difference in the way the world learns.

PART I

Background You Need

INTRODUCTION

Learning about the brain is no longer for scientists only. If you wanted to get your car fixed, you'd likely go to a mechanic. For legal help, you'd find an attorney. To understand the brain and how we learn, would you go to a teacher? Probably not. Yet every year, millions of parents trust that the professionals who teach their children know something about the brain and processes of learning. In defense of teachers, even neuroscientists still disagree on some of the inner workings of the brain. Many schools of education offer pop psychology but often not cognitive neuroscience or applied neurobiology courses. Inservice training is often directed at the symptoms of problems, not a working knowledge of the brain. Popular articles rarely offer the depth or point of view that today's educator needs. But this book will get you started in the field. How *I* got started is a bit unusual.

More than two decades ago, I got my first taste of "brain-compatible" learning. I took a course that was designed by facilitators who studied research on how our brain learns best. The impact was so powerful that even today, decades later, I could still fill up a flip chart page with ideas I remember (and still use!) from that workshop. The facilitators clearly understood some important principles about the brain. I became so enthusiastic (some would say a zealot) that I decided to share this excitement with others. Because I was teaching at that time, my first response was "Why don't my own students have this experience every day?" It was both humbling and promising.

This newfound brain-learning connection became my springboard for innovation. Soon after the workshop I cofounded an experimental, cutting-edge residential academic enrichment program called SuperCamp/ Quantum Learning. It became a global success, and the experiment we began years ago is now an international fixture with over 45,000 graduates. This program gave me a chance to see, hear, and feel the excitement from thousands of kids over the years. Kids who didn't like learning, school, or even themselves simply blossomed when put into a brain-compatible environment.

I am a zealot of brain-compatible teaching for a good reason. I have seen, felt, and heard firsthand the difference these learning principles make. Students of all backgrounds, with every imaginable history of failure, of every age and attitude of discouragement, can and have succeeded with this approach.

While this approach is not a panacea, it does provide some important directions as we move through the twenty-first century. Programs that are compatible with the way humans naturally learn will stand the test of time. Though brain-compatible teaching has been "proven" by teachers in real-world classrooms for years, it's gratifying to find that after years of research, the brain has now also made it onto the honored shelves of the academic elite.

This book is written for you—the classroom teacher, trainer, administrator, lifelong learner—you, a catalyst for doing the all-important work of facilitating learning the best way possible. The intent of this book is to introduce you to the basics of this exciting paradigm shift in education. If at the end you have a good grasp of the core differences between the traditional approach and the brain-compatible approach to learning, and a framework for understanding the principles presented, I will have satisfied my objective. If at the end you are also thinking, "Okay. . . . What's next?" I will be elated. For then I will have successfully passed on my passion for learning in a brain-compatible way. This should be the beginning of a transformational journey. Get ready for a great adventure!

—Eric Jensen

WHAT IS BRAIN-COMPATIBLE TEACHING?

Good question. Let's explore it a bit. The first form of schooling was simple. It was the apprenticeship method. For most of human history, if you wanted to learn about something, you'd find someone better at it than you and learn from him or her. This worked for centuries.

Then the industrial revolution hatched a new model. It was the notion that you could bring everyone together in a single place and offer a standardized, conveyor-belt curriculum. This second model or paradigm of schooling was developed in the 1800s and popularized through most of the twentieth century. It is often called the "factory model." Factory skills like obedience, orderliness, unity, and respect for authority were emphasized.

As we entered the information age in 1950 to today, there have been many models of how schools can and should work. Some are more traditional, focusing on controlling the flow of information and socialization. Others included the "demand model," "sage-on-the-stage," and "stand-and-deliver" models. Learners were expected to answer teacher questioning "on demand," and the teacher was considered the "expert" whose job it was to impart "knowledge" from the front of the classroom. But beginning in the early 1990s, a new model began to emerge.

A whole different breed of the science of teaching and learning was developing called educational neuroscience. It began as an exciting interdisciplinary approach to understanding the brain and was known as brain-compatible teaching.

> Brain-compatible learning is the understanding and teaching based on what we have learned *directly* from studying the brain. Brain-compatible teaching is the application of principles and strategies that *appear to be compatible* with what we know about the brain.

Brain-compatible teaching is the engagement of strategies based on principles of how our brain works in a school context. It will change our school start times, discipline policies, methods of assessment, teaching strategies, budget priorities, classroom environments, use of technology, and even the way we think of arts and physical education.

At first glance, brain-compatible teaching might seem like a lot of biology or principles that are mere platitudes on learning theory. But upon closer examination, educators are realizing that having hard science to support our successful classroom practices (ones we knew worked but were hard to prove) arms us with a greater degree of professionalism. The science of how the brain learns best is a revolution in learning—a transformation that will help us do a better job of reaching all students.

There are countless real-life personal and peer applications for the information in this book to ensure your success. You must try out these concepts for yourself, for it is in applying the learning that you will begin to fully understand brain-compatible learning. Once you experience it, the natural inclination is to want to share it with your students and colleagues.

When whole schools and districts have reassessed their thinking about learning, their curriculums, assessment methods, and school structures and have implemented brain-compatible strategies at this level, we will truly have reformed our educational institutions. Until we make research, reflection, and renewal as basic to schools as the three R's, our learning strategies will be less than optimal. As individual teachers, trainers, and administrators move toward the new paradigm, eventually everyone will benefit.

The following questions are addressed as you make your way through this guide.

- Does comparing one learner to another make sense?
- How are learners impacted by high stress and threat?
- How do windows of opportunity influence learners?
- When is it easiest to learn foreign languages?
- Why should fruit, protein, and nuts be in campus vending machines?
- Why are the phrases "on task" or "off task" irrelevant?
- Does the brain ever stop growing?
- What constitutes an enriched learning environment?
- How can we ensure students receive enough feedback?
- Why purposely engage strong emotions every day?
- Is no-stress learning the best kind?
- How can we get kids to remember more of what they learn?
- Why do kids tend not to pay attention in class?
- Why don't you want learners' attention most of the time?
- Why should school starting times be changed?
- Why post mind maps of whole units weeks in advance?
- Why is group work or cooperative learning good for the brain?
- To what degree does our brain change over time?
- In what ways does a brain-compatible curriculum boost student motivation?
- Why should rewards be eliminated from schools?

THE OLD AND NEW OF IT

OLD

Traditional approach
Behaviorist model
Control model
Reductionist thinking
Demand model
Sage on the stage
Hope based on. . . positive thinking
Identify goals for students
Comparison to others
Demand students learn
Stand and deliver
Reward desired behaviors
Punish negative behaviors

NEW

Understand key principles
Use the big picture/holistic thinking
Cooperative learning
Accept brain differences and treating them
Compare students only to their own prior work
Hope grounded in science
Focus on what drives positive change in the brain
Engage the rules for learning
Manage stress levels
Brain foods—enriched diets/glucose/hydration
Emotional readiness: safety, vesting, novelty, challenge, and goal
Input limitations/attention span limits
Sufficient settling time

WHEN BRAIN RESEARCH IS APPLIED TO THE CLASSROOM, EVERYTHING WILL CHANGE

- Discipline policies

  based on our biology and culture strengthening, not power/authority

- Curriculum

  developmentally appropriate and behaviorally and career relevant

- New teacher training

  teaching with the brain in mind, not test scores

- Classroom design

  better lighting, acoustics, temperature control

- Content per day/week/year

  less content/we would go much deeper with it

- Scheduling

  two school starting shifts/early bird (7:30 a.m.) and day bird (9:30 a.m.)

- Instructional strategies

  create safety, better vesting, add novelty, challenge, have input limitations, attention span limits, more activity, simulations, and experiential activities

- Assessment

  a portfolio on all, measure effort, love of learning, no high-stakes testing

- Budget priorities

  focus on prevention, pay teachers better, quality buildings

- Staff development

- Food service programs

- Technology

  no online classes until high school

- Bilingual programs

  better attention to culture, language, and time needed for ESL

- Special education

  better researched programs, more help, stronger long-term support

CHANGE CAN BE EASY!

Remember, dramatic change can come from

- Taking advantage of something you know about but don't do
- Eliminating something that's useless or harmful
- Being willing to "not know," to start over and learn anew
- Doing much more of something that you currently do

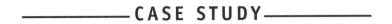
CASE STUDY

The 15-Year Change Process at an Elementary School

As principal of an elementary school in a high-poverty area, Dr. Matkin is focused on improving student assets through teacher quality. Many things have been part of the change process. First, everyone was involved in the decision making. Second, she has focused on changing attitudes as much as skill levels. Her school is in a high-poverty area, so she wanted every teacher to know, see, and believe that kids from poverty can learn well.

Third, she has made staff development a key part of the change process. Every new teacher gets the "brain-compatible" introduction, and she never lets up. She finds the funding to get every teacher trained. If they don't buy into the training over time, she'll encourage that teacher to find work elsewhere. Finally, she has been relentlessly positive. She is always focusing on the good in others and her students. While the district has tried to recruit her away from her school, she's stayed the course. She's taken her school from the bottom 25 percent to the top 25 percent in the state and a National Blue Ribbon School.

WE'RE NOT IN KANSAS ANYMORE

We need to be aware of the tendency to do things in a particular way just because that's the way we've always done them. But we also need to beware of the *"It's got to be new or it's not any good"* syndrome. As a new teacher, I did things the way my mentor teacher said. It was her way or no job. After 10 years, I realized that there are other, better ways to teach.

If pieces of the brain-compatible approach sound familiar to you, they are. But the pieces do not equal the available synergy. Avoid being lured into a false sense of familiarity. Teachers are creative and have tried thousands of strategies. Just because another teacher is using an idea that is promoted in this book, that does *not* mean they are "doing" brain-compatible teaching. Unless you know *why* you are using the strategy (the research behind it), you may drop a potentially powerful one only because you're bored with it. Brain-compatible teachers are purposeful. They can explain, with professionalism, the reason why they are using a strategy. As a result, they get more done, with less hit or miss.

It's not another fad; it's not ho-hum business as usual. This emerging field is nearly 30 years along. Taken as a whole, this approach provides a fundamentally different stage on which learning can be orchestrated.

WHERE'S THE PROOF?

Brain research can provide us with the specific studies that illuminate how our brain works. A cluster or aggregate of studies can provide us with a stronger, more generalizable principle. These principles can suggest a classroom strategy might be effective.

The Study

An example is the work of Dolcos and McCarthy (2006).

What I Found

Their results provide the very first direct brain-compatible evidence that details the negative effects of emotional distracters on ongoing cognitive processes. The study identifies the interactions within the frontal lobes between an upper neural system, associated with executive processing, and a lower system, associated with emotional processing. The brain underperforms with emotional distracters.

Is This the Only Study?

No, there are multiple other studies that suggest the potency of emotions and the susceptibility of the brain to emotional distracters.

What's the Principle?

Emotions can be a chronic negative force in the learning process.

What's the Potential Strategy?

Activities that either allow for the expression or the redirection of feelings may be helpful. Use the first few minutes of class time to allow for emotional processing and to steer emotions in a positive way. This might be accomplished through a walk, humor, partner time, positive social rituals, celebrations, reflection, sharing, or physical activities. Starting the class with content in the first five minutes may be counterproductive.

Notice the strategy suggested was not found in the research. Neuroscientists may not be good teachers. They don't suggest strategies. That comes from making the connections. Research on the brain does not necessarily "prove" that something is necessarily a good classroom strategy. That's too big a leap to make.

But the research can support and illuminate strategies already in use, steer us in the right direction, and help us avoid some highly inappropriate strategies. How can research do this? Scientists are paving this new ground with rapidly changing technological advances. Tomorrow's tools will be even more sophisticated, but here is a sampling of some common ones used currently.

TOOLS FOR EXPLORING THE BRAIN

FMRI (functional magnetic resonance imaging)

This tool provides high-quality cross-sectional images of soft tissue without X-rays or radiation.

Animals

Lab experiments done with rats, dogs, cats, slugs, apes, and others provide a rich source of information about how similar brains work. While some people are uncomfortable about animals being used for research, the government has established very strict standards that include housing conditions and food sources and that prohibit studies in which animals suffer. Many lab animals are treated better than household pets. We have learned a great deal about the human brain from studying the brains of animals.

Computerized electrodes (EEG and MEG)

These tools give readings about the electrical output of the brain. They've been used to detect brain wave patterns that represent various brain states and abnormal cerebral function such as seizures or dementia. These tools can also help us track, for example, how much activity is going on during problem solving.

Clinical studies

Using human volunteers, often from university psychology classes, we can learn much. For example, flashing slides at high speeds can tell us about reaction times of the visual system. Computer simulations can tell us much about decision making.

PET (positron emission tomography)

This imaging device tells us which areas are highly active. The subject is given an injection or drink of radioactive material with a short half-life (so it deteriorates quickly to safe levels) or radioactive glucose. Then it reads the amount of radioactive substances (positrons—the antimatter to electrons) released when certain areas of the brain consume glucose through usage.

Autopsies

The brain weight, stages of development, and amounts of decay, new cells, or lesions can all be observed or measured by a neurological pathologist. For example, using autopsies, University of California, Los Angeles neuroscientist Bob Jacobs discovered that students who had more challenging and demanding school lives had more dendritic branching (which some say represents a type of intelligence) than those who didn't.

Spectrometers

These devices measure the specifics of brain chemical movement as the activity is actually happening. For example, if I'm feeling depressed, a spectrometer measurement can tell me if there's been a change in the levels of specific neurotransmitters in my frontal lobes.

TEN REASONS TO CARE ABOUT BRAIN RESEARCH

10   Everybody has a brain, so this field includes everyone you work with and live with.

9   It's already talked about in the everyday news. More people are getting familiar with the research. There are several hundred journals and thousands of Internet sources that provide limitless data on the new research. You might as well join them and take advantage of what is known.

8   The new renaissance of brain research is now. This may be the most exciting time in human history to study the brain. You could personally meet the next da Vinci, Einstein, or Curie.

7   It can help you get ahead in life. You could learn new things, become much smarter, or have a better memory. It could help you avoid brain injury or recover faster from one.

6   The brain is 2 percent of your body's weight but uses 20 percent of your body's energy. Shouldn't you know where all that energy goes?

5   It can make your job easier as you find out how to be much more efficient by doing the right things in class instead of getting frustrated and having to reteach often.

4   Discover some really useful things: how to improve your memory, stay focused, lower your stress at work, and even how to boost learning for school or personal reasons.

3   You are losing thousands of brain cells every day and generating some brand new ones (it's called neurogenesis) too. Find out what to do so that you can end the day with a net gain of brain cells.

2   It can be quite practical. Find out why some students don't learn as well as others and learn what to do about it. Discover the secrets of learning delays, dyslexia, agraphia, autism, or dyscalculia.

1   We will *all* get old someday. The older you live, the greater the likelihood of diseases like dementia, Alzheimer's, or Parkinson's. You can learn how to prevent or even treat them.

THE EVOLUTION OF BRAIN MODELS

Primitive models on the workings of the brain have been around for 2,000 years. Each of these models fit with the times and often used the most exciting or pervasive technology as a metaphor.

Going back 2,000 years, the brain was referred to as a hydraulic system (the Greco-Roman model). By the 1700s, it was a fluid system (Renaissance), then an enchanted loom in the 1800s (the early industrial revolution). More recently, it was referred to as (no surprise here) a city's switchboard (early to mid-1900s) and, in the last half-century, yes, the amazing computer (1950s to recent).

The split-brain theory (Roger Sperry) of the 1970s told us that we just needed more right-brain or whole-brain learning. Karl Pribram's holographic model (1980s) said everything was everywhere else too in the brain. The holographic model was another example of technology as the brain model. Richard Restak's modular brain theory (late 1980s) said our brain has many compartments and modules and that each one could explain our behaviors. This reductionist model said that if you could isolate any individual part of the brain, you could understand its value to the system. It studies parts, not wholes. As an example, our emotional responses were isolated in the amygdala, so that must be what guides our emotions. Today we know it's much more complex.

The triune brain theory (originated in 1952 and popularized in the 1990s) introduced the three-part evolutionary-based schema that told us survival learning was in the lower brain, emotions were in the midbrain, and higher-order thinking was in the upper-brain area. This model was so simple, and that made it quite attractive. But our current understanding is more complex.

The current model may be closest to the holographic brain model, but it's more literal. It espouses that every structure in the brain has some relational connectivity (physical, chemical, electrical, or peripheral) to another. This model embraces the body-mind as a second circuit for information exchange. The peptides (amino acids) found throughout the body are just as important for information exchange as the brain's other system of neuronal connectivity—synapses. It says that the brain is dynamic and changing every single day.

In short, the days of asking, What does this part of the brain do? are diminishing. We now know that the brain's functioning often depends on the specific situation, emotions present at the time, the age of individuals, their health, and their past experiences. We are realizing just how complex the brain really is!

BE A BRAIN-SMART CONSUMER: RECOGNIZING GOOD RESEARCH

Clinical Studies

Clinical studies are usually university supported, preferably with multiple experimenters, double-blind design, and large, diverse, multiage, multicultural populations. They try out an idea that may need strict controls to ensure validity. This study was conducted at the University of California, Irvine.

An example was the studies done to introduce, disprove, or prove the "Mozart Effect." The original study was done by Rauscher, Shaw, Levine, Ky, and Wright (1993). Since this initial study, over 30 others have attempted to replicate, enhance, or move beyond the "music and intelligence" debate.

"In Context" Studies

Done in schools, this documented action research gives us testing results under actual, real-life conditions. An example is Huttenlocher, Levine, and Vevea (1998). This study found a positive correlation between school language input and cognitive growth in a single population of children.

Basic Neuroscience: The Discovery Studies

This is the hard science department. It could come from autopsies, experiments, FMRI, PET, or EEG scans. This should get your interest, but it's not the final word. Look for multiple studies to support an idea. A groundbreaking study done by Eriksson et al. (1998) showed that humans can and do grow new brain cells. Amazingly, later studies showed that our everyday behaviors could regulate this process.

Brain Theory (Be cautious; this is not actual research)

These are any models about learning and the brain that explain that recurring behaviors may be overly simplistic. Famous people usually make up theories, but they might not be true. Examples include the triune or holographic brain theories. A theory is sometimes very attractive; it's an idea that can become popular, even though unproven.

ACTION OR THEORY: WHO WANTS TO READ ALL THAT RESEARCH?

Yes, it can get a bit technical—especially when they're talking about post-traumatic lesions in the anterior medial temporal lobe resulting in retrograde amnesia. Aaaargh! But relax. You don't have to know all these words.

First, there's only a small percentage of brain research that carries with it useful applications for educators. Much of it is highly detailed, theoretical, or pathology (disease) oriented. Brain research isn't usually directed at traditional learning; however, it can suggest ideas or educational paths that have a higher probability of success. A great deal of action or applied research in the classroom is still needed. A great deal of what's useful and what's not will come from thoughtful educators like yourself who take the lab research concept seriously and turn it into action research.

Second, there are a limited number of principles that make up the brain-compatible teaching paradigm. When applied correctly, these principles will revolutionize learning and education. Yet, it's not how much you know about the brain that matters, it's how much you apply!

Take what you learn and experiment with it. Keep a journal, reflect, share, dialogue, consider feedback, and correct. You don't need a pile of scholarly research (although much of it is very interesting!) to make a big difference in your students' lives. As a country, we do more educational research than any other country in the world and we ignore more of it as well. It is the action or application of the research that we need in our classrooms, not theory. With the basic knowledge you are acquiring right now, you will be equipped to apply the research.

The rate at which you learn will become the only sustainable competitive advantage you'll have in your life.

—Peter Senge

EXCELLENT SOURCES OF RESEARCH

American Journal of Occupational Therapy

Biological Psychiatry

Brain and Behavior

Brain in the News (Dana Press)

Brain Research

Cerebrum (Dana Press)

Developmental Psychology

Developmental Psychobiology

Early Childhood Research Quarterly

Early Education and Development

Exceptional Children

Journal of Abnormal Child Psychology

Journal of Applied Developmental Psychology

Journal of Behavioral Education

Journal of Cognitive Neuroscience

Journal of Early Intervention

Journal of Emotional and Behavioral Disorders

Journal of Neurobiology

Journal of Neuroscience

Journal of Pediatric Psychology

Journal of Special Education

Language, Speech and Hearing Services in Schools

Learning and the Brain

Neuroscience and Behavioral Physiology

Occupational Therapy Journal of Research

Proceedings of the National Academy of Sciences of the United States of America

Public Medical Library ("PubMed") online searches

List of Brainy Web Sites

www.sciencedaily.com/news/mind_brain.htm

www.dana.org/books/press

schoolstudio.engr.wisc.edu/brainbased.html

FUN FACTOIDS ON THE BRAIN

3 and 1,350	The number of pounds and grams, respectively, that the adult human brain weighs
17 and 7,800	The number of pounds and grams, respectively, that the adult sperm whale brain weighs
7	The percentage that the average male brain is larger in size than the average female brain
7	The percentage that the average male body size is larger than the female
4	The average weight, in pounds, of a dolphin brain
1	The average weight, in pounds, of a gorilla brain
540	The average number of square inches of the "unfolded" human cortex
4	The number of lobes of the human brain
1 million	The number of nerve fibers in the adult human brain
13–15	The age, in years, that the average corpus callosum is fully myelinated
1	The number of synaptic connections between our nose and the amygdala
100	Speed, in meters per second, of the fastest neural transmissions
2	The average percentage of your own brain's weight versus your body weight
78	The average percentage of water, by weight, that the human brain is made of
6	The number of different layers in the cerebral cortex
1 trillion	The estimated number of glia (support cells) in a human brain

2	The estimated percentage of the brain-body communication that occurs at the synaptic level (the rest is through widely dispersed peptide molecules)
100 billion	The number of neurons in an average adult brain
50 billion	The known quantity of types of chemical messengers (neurotransmitters) identified so far
10	The average percentage of fat, by weight, that the human brain is made of
8	The average percentage of protein, by weight, that the human brain is made of
0.25	The thickness, in inches, of our neocortex
1 trillion	Typical number of connections in a newborn's brain
50 trillion	The number of synaptic connections in an adult's brain

WHAT'S IN THE HUMAN BRAIN?

Our brain consists of water, proteins, fat, tissue, and plenty of sophisticated structures. Scientists divide the brain into four areas called lobes. They are occipital, frontal, parietal, and temporal.

Frontal (judgment, creativity, decision making, planning).

This is the "parent voice" or voice of authority.

Parietal (higher sensory, spatial, short-term memory).

This is the circus of the brain with capacity for the trapeze artists.

Temporal (language, writing, hearing, sensory associations, explicit memory).

This is the digital recorder or TiVo in the brain, recording the most requested or relevant "shows" from life experiences.

Occipital (receives and processes visual information).

This is the videocam in the brain, recording what you see.

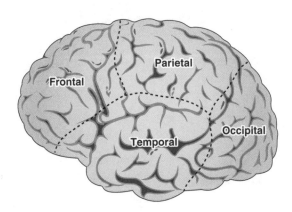

The occipital lobe is in the middle back of the brain. It's primarily responsible for vision. The frontal lobe is the area around your forehead. It's involved with purposeful acts like judgment, creativity, problem solving, and planning. The parietal lobe is on the top back area. Its duties include processing sensory, motor, and spatial functions. The temporal lobes (left and right side) are above and around the ears. These areas are primarily responsible for hearing, memory, meaning, and language. There is some overlap in the functions of the lobes.

BRAIN TEASER

Draw the four lobes of the brain below without looking back on the previous page. (This will strengthen your learning.)

THE BRAIN DIVIDED

Right-Left Hemispheres

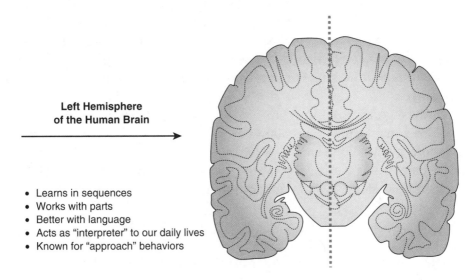

Left Hemisphere of the Human Brain

- Learns in sequences
- Works with parts
- Better with language
- Acts as "interpreter" to our daily lives
- Known for "approach" behaviors

The Brain Has Two Hemispheres

They are covered by a sheet of wrinkled skin called the neocortex (a ¼-inch-thick wrinkled skinlike tissue).

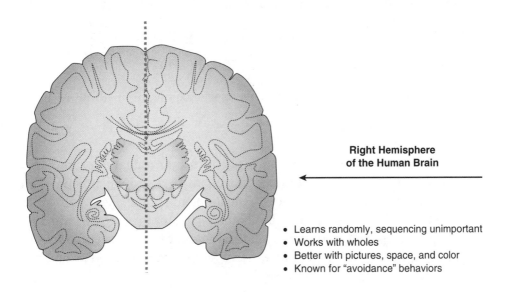

Right Hemisphere of the Human Brain

- Learns randomly, sequencing unimportant
- Works with wholes
- Better with pictures, space, and color
- Known for "avoidance" behaviors

THE BRAIN CONNECTED

The corpus callosum is a bundle of nerve tissue (about 250 million nerves) connecting the left- and right-brain hemispheres. It serves as the Golden Gate Bridge (or Brooklyn Bridge) for connections and functioning. Patients in whom the corpus callosum has been severed can still function in society. However, they have difficulty connecting language and thoughts, words and pictures, and making common associations that you and I likely take for granted.

On average, the callosum connection is thicker in women, with 20 million more fibers than in men. This allows each hemisphere to exchange information more freely. While each side of the brain does process things differently, some of our earlier assumptions about the left-right brain split are outdated now. Here is what we know about which side does what:

Our brain's left hemisphere processes information more sequentially.

Musicians commonly process music in their left hemisphere.

A novice would probably process music on the right side.

Nearly half of left handers use their right hemisphere for language.

Higher-level mathematicians, problem solvers. and chess players have more right hemisphere activation during those activities.

Beginners in those activities usually are more left-hemisphere active.

Gross motor function is controlled by the right hemisphere.

Fine motor is usually more left-hemisphere activity.

The right hemisphere is where we experience negative emotions.

Our left hemisphere is more active as we have positive emotions.

Sometimes the hemisphere we use changes over time. For example, in infants, some of the earliest language processing is right hemisphere. Then by age three and four, it has moved to the left hemisphere. Females tend to develop their left hemisphere earlier than males. This gives them a distinct advantage in language and reading skills. Males are superior to females in right-hemisphere development at age five, but both sexes even out by age eight or nine. Males tend to become more right hemisphere as they grow past age 50 into their older years.

Suffice it to say that the old biases about music and arts being "right-brain frills" are outdated. We do have real *preferences*, but those are different than being exclusively left or right brained. All of us have noticed that some people are often more sequential and others more global/random. So while it's accurate to talk of preferences, it's not accurate to talk about left-right absolutes.

BRAIN GEOGRAPHY

The middle or "medial" brain is the region behind the frontal lobes and in front of the occipital lobe. This term represents a *geographical* location. The commonly used term "limbic brain" refers also to the midbrain area, but it represents a *functional* location in the brain.

The limbic area defines the part of the brain that processes, among other tasks, our emotions. Much of the middle of the brain area is not involved in processing emotions. That's the role of many other processes diversified in our brain and body. Here is a description of some of the key structures located in the brain's center:

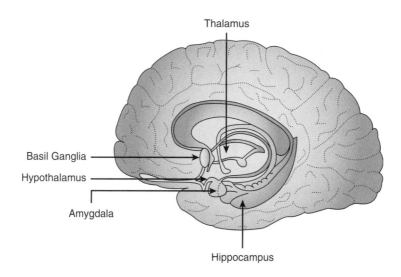

Thalamus

The thalamus is the sorting station for most sensory input. It's a bit like the Web server for a domain name. It's a router of information, going in both directions. All new sensory input (except smell) goes to our thalamus first before it goes to other areas of the brain.

Hypothalamus

The hypothalamus is located below the thalamus; it's the brain's thermostat that regulates body functions. It operates on feedback and feed forward from the environmental signals. It both learns from them and anticipates what will happen next. In fact, it's a system that responds to a measured change in a predefined way to maintain stability.

Basil Ganglia

The basil ganglia is an important area responsible for smooth motor functions. When this area does not get sufficient or accurate input, we become clumsy.

Amygdala

The amygdala is an almond-shaped structure located low in the middle of the brain. It is highly survival-oriented and processes suspicion, fear, and uneasiness as well as other intense emotions. Think of its role as something like a smoke detector for your brain. It becomes most activated with uncertainty and risk. While it can activate very, very, fast, it can also operate like a dimmer switch at times. Like a smoke detector, it does give us false alarms, preferring to alert us too often rather than ignoring a potentially harmful threat. As a result, we may become scared, reacting to a rustle in the bushes, even if it's a rabbit (not a thug). But that's better than underreacting!

Hippocampus

The hippocampus is a crescent-shaped structure curving from the top to the bottom of the middle of the brain. It's responsible for the formation of explicit long-term memories. In many ways, it acts like a surge protector, preventing too much information getting into long-term storage. Once past the working memory, new learning is stored in the hippocampus as a layover depot before being moved to long-term storage.

Brain Stem

The brain stem includes the pons, which regulates facial sensations and movements, and the medulla, which regulates and relays many nonconscious operations like heartbeat, breathing, and digestion.

Cerebellum

The cerebellum (or "little brain" in Greek) is located near the brain stem, below the occipital lobe. It is involved in posture, coordination, balance, motor memory, plus counting, ordering, and other cognitive activities. It's a bit like the gyroscope in the brain keeping you level and balanced.

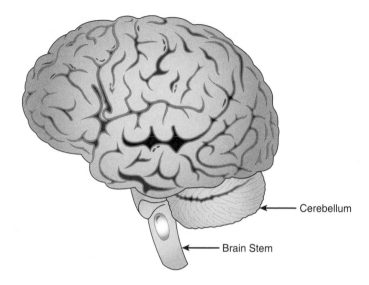

Cerebellum

Brain Stem

The cerebellum, an area most commonly linked to movement, turns out to be a virtual switchboard of cognitive activity. The cerebellum takes up just 1/10 of the brain by volume but contains almost half of all the brain's total neurons. It has some 40 million nerve fibers, 40 times more than even the highly complex optical tract. These fibers not only feed information from the cortex to the cerebellum, but they feed them back to the cortex. If the cerebellum were only for motor function (as was once thought), why would the connections be so powerfully distributed in both directions to all areas of the brain? This subsection of the brain, long known for its role in posture, balance, ordering, rhythm, and movement, may be our brain's sleeping giant.

BRAIN "CELL"EBRATION: FAR-OUT FACTS ABOUT BRAIN CELLS

You have nearly 1 trillion brain cells! There are two kinds of brain cells: neurons and glia. Though the majority of brain cells (85–90 percent) are glia, the remaining 10–15 percent are the neurons. A huge amount of the brain's information transfer happens through the cell-to-cell process. When stimulated, brain cells grow branchlike extensions called dendrites. Each cell has one extending leg called an axon. The axons can grow up to a meter long. They often subdivide many times. Only axons connect with dendrites; dendrites don't connect with other dendrites.

Neurons will typically make 1,000 to 50,000 connections with other neurons. We are born with more connections than we'll need, but we lose about half of our brain's connections by age 12. A typical brain has well over a trillion connections.

Here are 10 key facts about your brain's inner workings:

1 New research suggests we can and do grow new brain cells or neurons (Eriksson et al., 1998). Fred Gage at the Salk Institute of Biological Studies in San Diego, California, led the research team.

2 Neurons don't sleep. A normal functioning neuron is continuously firing, integrating, and generating information; it's a virtual hotbed of activity. What changes with environmental input is the intensity and pattern of firing.

3 No neuron is an end point or termination for information; it only serves to pass it on. All electrical activity in the brain travels from the receiving dendrites to the neural body (soma), then down to the axon (output).

4 A single neuron may connect through its dendrites with countless other cells. This is a good sign; the more the connections your cells make, the better. Genes, enrichment, and its specific location determine how many connections a neuron makes with other connections. Cells in the cerebellum have the greatest dendritic branching.

5 The sum total of all the synaptic reactions arriving from all the dendrites to the cell body at any moment will determine whether that cell will, in fact, fire. It needs a "majority vote." In other words, learning is the critical function of neurons that cannot be accomplished individually—it requires groups of neurons.

6 Most adult neuronal bodies stay put; they simply extend an axon outward. While many fibers (dendrites) may extend from a neuron, each neuron has only one axon. An axon is a thinner, leglike extension that connects to dendrites.

7 The axon has two essential functions: to conduct information in the form of electrical stimulation and to transport chemical substances. The longest ones may be up to a meter long (spinal cord). The thicker the axons, the faster it conducts electricity (and information).

8 Myelin is a lipid (fatty) substance that forms around well-used axons. The most used neurons are myelinated. This seems not only to speed up the electrical transmission (up to twelvefold) but also to reduce interference from other nearby reactions.

9 The point of contact between two neurons is the synapse. It's a micro gap where the electrical nerve impulse traveling down the axon triggers the release of chemical messengers (neurotransmitters) stored at the end of the axon. The receptor sites in the connecting dendrites absorb them.

10 The synapse is the point of communication for less than 2 percent of the body's total communication. The rest of it comes from the floating information bundles known as peptides, which lock into receptor sites and transfer data through absorption.

LEARNING HAPPENS . . . BUT HOW?

Scientists are unsure exactly how humans learn, but they have some ideas about the likely process. For what we call explicit learning (names, facts, pictures, text, etc.), the process is a bit challenging to list because it's not 100 percent sequential. Many processes are happening in parallel, some on a micro, others on a macro level. It may go like this:

A Stimulus to the Brain Starts the Process

It could be internal (a brainstorm!) or it could be a new experience, like solving a jigsaw puzzle. Novel mental or motor stimulation activates what we call input neurons located in our tactile, olfactory, auditory, or visual areas. These input neurons are stimulated and send their signals to the thalamus.

The Thalamus Directs the Signals

The thalamus sends signals to multiple areas of the brain for further processing. Visual input will go to the occipital area. At the same time, temporary representations of the information may be sent to our working memory (located in frontal lobes for visual and parietal/temporal lobes for auditory processing). Simultaneously, information is being sent through the amygdala.

The Amygdala Gets an Inside Track and Quick Read

To ensure survival, the amygdala gets first crack at all information to determine if there are any "survival issues." An object thrown at you, a siren, slippery walkway, loaded gun, or child's cry will be processed immediately, before other detailed information. If appropriate, this structure will activate signals in the hypothalamus that starts the alarm response. Otherwise, this structure stays less active.

Activity Hits the Middle Layers of Neurons

Once the activity moves beyond the "input" neurons, it'll go through many other layers of neurons for processing. The visual system alone has over 15 layers (e.g., movement, color, contrast). Once these areas process the new input, we create aggregates of the raw data called rough drafts.

Rough Drafts Are Commonplace

From our working memory, these rough drafts will emerge *if* we remain interested in the new learning. The temporary representation of new learning is usually a bit sketchy. It may not be accurate, clear, or complete. These rough drafts are stored in the hippocampus.

The Hippocampus Is a "Layover Depot"

Our two hippocampi are located in the temporal lobes. They're small C-shaped structures that learn fast but have a small memory capacity. They simply cannot store very much information. They hold the temporary representations, or rough drafts, until we either drop them or make them more meaningful or somehow worth saving. Some new learning may stay in the hippocampi for days. Eventually, the hippocampi will send the information packages to the cortex.

The Cortex Saves Many of Our Memories

We store many types of memories. The more explicit ones (pictures, names, facts, etc.) are stored in the ¼-inch layer that covers our lobes. These lobes store the same type of information that they originally processed. The visual cortex processes *and* stores visual components of our memories.

Formation of a Memory Potential

Learning is regulated by both genetics and life experience. Once the cell signals are activated, a switch known as CREB (cAMP reactive elemental binding) signals the neuron to activate either short- or long-term memory. A gene is responsible for activating the protein formation for long-term memory. If a weaker stimulus is then applied to the neighboring cell sometime later, the cell's ability to get excited is enhanced. In other words, cells change their receptivity to messages based on previous stimulation. This lasting learning or LTP (long-term potentiation) is tentatively accepted by most scientists as the physical process that stores learning.

Let's Review

At the micro level, when neurons connect at the synapse, the connection goes from electrical to chemical to electrical. This junction point (the synapse) becomes stronger (synaptic adhesion), and the two neurons can talk to each other with much less signal needed. On the macro level, input neurons send signals through our thalamus, working memory, and then our hippocampus, where they may be sent to the cortex for long-term storage.

ARE TODAY'S KIDS DIFFERENT?

Unless you compared hundreds of saved brains (not done) or actual brain scans (not available 30 years ago), you would not know for sure if today's kids are different. However, the evidence suggests that kids today have different brains. Why? Two simple facts: (1) the brain changes as a result of experience and (2) experiences are different for today's kids contrasted with those of two generations ago.

Change in Diet

Today, kids maintain a higher fat, sugar, and carbohydrates diet with fewer proteins. Foods can impact the functioning, but not usually the structure, of the brain (heavy alcohol causes brain atrophy). This may significantly change the brain. Some studies point not only to the impact of poor diets on the children but to the potential long-term effects through the cellular capacity for gene expression (Fox, Pac, Devaney, & Jankowski, 2004; Kilberg, Pan, Chen, & Leung-Pineda, 2005; Mahoney, Lord, & Carryl, 2005; Pollitt, Gorman, Engle, Rivera, & Martorelli, 1995).

Drug and Medication Usage

Blurred lines exist between drugs and medications. More kids are willing to take something to alter their mind and body states. While the use of traditional drugs (heroin, cocaine, alcohol, and marijuana) has declined slightly, other problems have risen. From 1992 to 2002, new abuse of prescription opioids among 12- to 17-year-olds was up an astounding 542 percent, more than 4 times the rate of increase among adults. In 2003, 2.3 million 12- to 17-year-olds (nearly 1 in 10) abused at least one controlled prescription drug; for 83 percent of them, the drug was opioids. Kids today use many prescription drugs obtained from their parents or peers (for allergies, ADHD, and other maladies) and even more nonprescribed medications (Oxycontin, Vicodin, Valium, etc.) compared to 30 years ago. Teens who abuse controlled prescription drugs are twice as likely to use alcohol, 5 times likelier to use marijuana, 12 times likelier to use heroin, 15 times likelier to use Ecstasy, and 21 times likelier to use cocaine, compared to teens who do not abuse such drugs (National Center on Addiction and Substance Abuse at Columbia University, 2005).

Less "Crawl Time" and Physical Activity

We are in cars more than ever. Infants are becoming "bucket babies," going from car seats to high chairs to cribs with little opportunity for exploratory play. Poor motor development is being impacted by (a) an increase in the amount of inactive time spent in automobiles, watching television, and in front of computers, (b) the disappearance of swings, seesaws, and merry-go-rounds, (c) a reduction in school physical education programs, and (d) a lack of emphasis on walking or riding bikes versus motorized transportation. Evidence suggests we are in cars more, yet those who explore more become more intelligent (Carter, 1999; Hu & Young, 1999; Raine, Reynolds, Venables, & Mednick, 2002; U.S. Department of Transportation, Bureau of Transportation Statistics, 2006).

Social/Economic Stability

Many children are growing up with fewer resources. In 1960, over 90 percent of all unwed mothers gave up their baby for adoption to qualified families. Today, over 90 percent of all unwed mothers keep their babies, in spite of a lack of financial, health, or emotional resources. This is a significant turnaround with profound effects (Fields & Casper, 2001; U.S. Census Bureau, 1998).

School Budget Cuts

Fewer music, drama, and arts classes are available in public schools today. As resources tighten, the arts are often considered a right-brained frill. Many decision makers know better, but not all, and in the midst of competing agendas, the arts are wrongly considered nonessential. The absence of arts and physical education may be changing the brain (Fiske, 1999).

Less Close Family Time

Children today are more likely to be raised by a combination of caregivers. Over 60 percent will have spent a significant amount of time in child care, compared to just 10 percent two generations ago. This lack of emotional stability and attunement development often changes the brain. It may create hyper and hypo responsiveness to daily stressors (Ramey & Ramey, 2000; Schore, 2000).

The Increasingly Violent Digital World

There is more exposure today to video games and TV with threat, stress, and violence. More kids are impacted by excess violence on television than ever before and by violence in their homes, schools, and communities. The evidence for correlations is stronger between digital violence and real-life violence than it is for secondhand smoke or global warming, both highly accepted positions (Anderson & Bushman, 2001; Joy, Kimball, & Zabrack, 1986).

More Hours of Media Per Week

The average child is watching media three to five hours per day (20–30 hours per week). Excessive television viewing leads to greater passivity, antisocial behavior, and less thinking time. Too many kids are learning about the world secondhand! Some concern exists regarding the impact of TV on the developmental stages of children. Others believe that excess attention to a fast-moving media is part of the problem for today's short attention-span kids (Christakis, Zimmerman, DiGiuseppe, & McCarty, 2004; Johnson, Cohen, Smailes, Kasen, & Brook, 2002; Murray, 1994; Rideout & Vandewater, 2003; Strasburger & Donnerstein, 2000).

BOYS' AND GIRLS' BRAIN DIFFERENCES

The descriptions below generalize what neuroscientists typically call an average "female" or average "male" brain. Keep in mind that they are based on statistical averages, and that in real life, *there can be major variances* in hormone levels, behaviors, and brain structures. While there is some overlap in these two bell-shaped statistical profiles, they are largely different.

Female Brain

- Develops the left hemisphere earlier than the right
- Has a larger corpus callosum (3–10 percent more fibers) than male
- Has monthly fluctuations in the two hormones progesterone and estrogen, which causes shifting scores on spatial, math, verbal, and fine motor skills tests (lower hormone levels result in a boost in scores on spatial and math tests; higher hormone levels result in a boost in verbal and fine motor skills)
- Has 20–30 percent more serotonin, which is correlated with fearfulness, shyness, lower self-confidence, and unduly dampened aggression
- Spreads thinking function over a wider area of the brain, which translates to fewer learning disabilities
- Performs better at things that require multitasking
- Responds more to soothing words and song
- Often displays dampened aggression, more covert negative behaviors
- Can distinguish faces and photos earlier and better
- Seeks survival alliances with friends based more on relationships than utility
- Has higher baseline of estrogen, for better verbal and fine motor skills
- Can identify the emotional content of speech easier
- Has more brain traffic between left and right hemispheres

Male Brain

- Develops the right hemisphere earlier than in females, which impacts classroom discipline and preferences in sports
- Maintains higher testosterone levels, which aid skills in abstract manipulation, spatial, science, math, and sports. High levels are detrimental to these fields.

- Is more compartmentalized and less distributed in functional areas than in females
- Has 20–30 percent less serotonin; this lower level is correlated with impulsive aggression, suicide, alcoholism, and explosive rage
- Learns to speak and read later than females
- Has a left hemisphere that develops later than the right
- Is more specialized, with more modular learning in brain—more learning disabilities
- Processes emotional events in wholes, not in sequenced parts
- Has less interest in communication with others, more in things and processes
- Displays less fearfulness and shyness and shows higher self-confidence
- Matures in the frontal lobes later than other areas of the brain
- Has more behavior preservation; less flexible, but better at maintaining new habits (Cahill, Uncapher, Kilpatrick, Alkire, & Turner, 2004; Coffey et al., 1998; Collins & Kimura, 1997; Davatzikos & Resnick, 1998; Delgado & Prieto, 1996; Harasty, Double, Halliday, Kril, & McRitchie, 1997; Killgore, Oki, & Yurgelun-Todd, 2001; Pomerantz, Altermatt, & Saxon, 2002; Schlaepfer et al., 1995; Witelson, Glezer, & Kigar, 1995)

LEARNING DISABILITIES: DIFFERENT BRAINS

Though learning conditions are often lumped into one large soup bowl called disabilities, each student needs to be carefully and independently diagnosed. Remember, differences do not equal disabilities. An accurate diagnosis will start the process to a more effective response and treatment. Here are some examples of those with learning difficulties.

Reading Problems

These are sometimes the result of the brain just not being ready to read (maturity). Boys mature later than girls in the left (the reading) hemisphere. Give them a bit more time. Reading problems can be visual (poor acuity, poor tracking or depth perception). Reading difficulties may also be a result of poor phonological processing (they can't separate the phonemes, such as being able to know that *cat* is *cuh-aah-tih*). In addition, they may have problems in poor vocabulary, text comprehension, or fluency. Only proper diagnosis and committed interventions will get these students back on board.

Learning Delays

The number one cause of students' inability to make the usual developmental milestones is fetal alcohol exposure. But learning delays may also come from prenatal stress, exposure to toxins, brain injury, abuse, or neglect. Typically, these students have speech and language impairments, they are poor at linking up cause and effect, and have weak memory. Their brain's primary difficulty is that neurons are not as well connected as they should be. Learning takes more meaning, more trial and error, and certainly more repetitions for these students. They can also use enrichment as much as anyone.

Attention-Deficit/Hyperactivity Disorder

ADHD has become a catchword for a variety of behaviors that can be the result of genetic predisposition, head trauma, compromised neural pathways, or neurotransmitter (serotonin/dopamine) irregularities. Symptoms include a sluggish brain, impulsivity, poor short-term memory, prolonged restlessness, and inability to plan ahead or reflect on the past. Drug intervention ought to be a last resort. Other interventions like a change of diet, increased physical activity, changing teachers, or teacher accommodations or special success strategies should be made first.

Asperger's

This condition is found at the more functional end of the wide range of autistic spectrum disorders. While severe autism may strike as few as 1 in 10,000, Asperger's may strike as often as 1 in 160. This condition is most commonly characterized by poor social skills, repetitive behaviors, difficulty in changing plans or routines, and sensory difficulties. Students with this disorder may have average or above average IQ. However, there is a wide range of behavioral possibilities; make no assumptions about capacity or symptoms. With successful interventions, these students may be able to function quite well.

THE CRANIAL SOUP BOWL: UNDERSTANDING THE CHEMICALS IN OUR BRAINS

Four Common Neurotransmitters

Neurotransmitters are our brain's best-known biochemical messengers. We have about 50 of them. They are the stimulus or the inhibitors that regulate neural activity.

Acetylcholine

Acetylcholine is a common neurotransmitter, particularly involved in long-term memory formation. Specifically released at neuromuscular junctions, it's present at higher levels during sleep. It is needed to form memories.

Dopamine (it's the "yahoo" chemical)

Dopamine is a powerful and common neurotransmitter primarily involved in producing a positive mood or feelings. Synthesized by proteins and secreted by specialized neurons in the substantia nigra, midbrain, and hypothalamus, it plays a role in movements and working memory. Dopamine deficits are found in patients suffering from Parkinson's disease.

GABA (it's the "eeee-eekkk" or brake pedals in the brain)

Gamma-aminobutyric acid is a neurotransmitter that acts as an inhibitory agent—an off switch in the brain. All learning requires just the right combination of neural activity (excitatory chemicals) and neural suppression (inhibitory chemicals). Without GABA, you'd have too much neural activity, and seizures would result.

Serotonin (it's the feeling mellow or "ahhhh" feeling)

Serotonin is a common neurotransmitter, most responsible for inducing relaxation and regulating mood and sleep. Males average about 20 to 30 percent less than females. Serotonin affects learning, attention, sleep, arousal, and memory. It increases behavioral and cognitive flexibility—just the right amount is good, too much makes us fearful, lacking self-confidence, and obsessive-compulsive. Too little is correlated with aggression and depression.

PART II

The Foundation for Teaching Is Principles, Not Strategies

WHAT ARE THE PRINCIPLES?

Principle 1: The Principle of Change: Brain Is Dynamic, Not Fixed

This means that no matter what are the levels of frustration or low achievement or even behavioral problems, the brain has the capacity to change.

Principle 2: The Principle of Variety: All Brains Are Unique

This strengthens the notion that there's no one-size-fits-all style of teaching, environment, curriculum, or assessment. We must continually find ways to match what we do with our learners.

Principle 3: The Principle of Developmental Sensitivity

At different ages, we have different vulnerabilities and possibilities. We could characterize the sensitive and vulnerable periods as the following: (a) prenatal, (b) birth to 5, (c) 5 to 12, and (c) 12 to 18. There are both risks and opportunities at each of those periods that should not be ignored.

Principle 4: The Principle of Interaction: We Have a "Social Brain"

Humans will not develop successfully in isolation. Our culture provides signals for emotional development, cultural standards, and social behaviors. We would be wise to consider the context, the social environment at school, as an area of huge risk and opportunity.

Principle 5: The Principle of Connectivity: The Brain Is an Integrated "System of Systems"

This principle reminds us that anything that is going on in one area of our life may influence another. This means we should pay extra attention to the role of nutrition, distress, chronic pain, drug abuse, lack of exercise, depression, trauma, and any other home life or school variable as potentially influencing the learning.

Principle 6: The Principle of Memory Malleability

The old belief was that memories are like photographs and that they are stored intact, lasting for some time. We now know that memories are actually a collection of properties (location, day of the week, who was there, what was said, how you felt, what you wore, the smells, etc.). These properties only rarely get reactivated all at the time of retrieval, but they are highly subject to alteration, decay, and bias. In short, most memories are not very reliable.

Principle 7: The Principle of Resource Consumption

There are structural limitations, physical processes, and resources that get consumed in the learning process. These place some guidelines and limitations on what gets learned and how much gets learned. When you know what enhances and what limits the learning, you can influence the variables to optimize every student's potential.

NOTE: We could formulate more principles that would be more specific. We could even consolidate these into fewer principles. What is important is that the upcoming principles are accurate, manageable, and practical.

PRINCIPLE 1: THE PRINCIPLE OF CHANGE: BRAIN IS DYNAMIC, NOT FIXED

Years ago, educators thought younger kids had smaller brains and we filled them up with knowledge and skills. We now know that the brain is constantly changing. What is it that changes? Nearly everything!

- The size, shape, and quantity of cells
- The number of new connections
- The levels of brain chemicals
- The pattern of neural activity
- The amount of mass in brain areas

The old paradigm was that our genes are simply the blueprints that make copies called RNA (ribonucleic acid, which is a "messenger and copy" molecule) involved in cell replication. Yet we have only about 25,000 genes. Our complexity cannot come only from genes; we share 70 percent of the same genes as a pumpkin! Even chimpanzees share 98 percent of the same genes as humans! Just for comparison, a chicken and a spotted puffer fish also have about 25,000 genes. Where on earth does all the human complexity come from? But what if genes did more than make copies? It turns out that they do!

Our new understanding is that genes have not one, but two functions. One is to replicate themselves through RNA. The other, more amazing function is to be responsive to environmental signals. This process is called gene expression. The 2006 Nobel Prize in physiology went to a pair of scientists who described this process and how to influence it in a laboratory. Alterations in what the organism considers status quo will influence the expression of genes by altering their messages to proteins. Factors such as stress, nutrition, exercise, social factors, trauma, and even extended emotional states can influence gene expression. This new discovery explains many so-called miracles in education, the ones we simply never thought would happen (Rossi, 2002).

If the interactions are positive and sustained, you'll get one set of changes. If the interactions are negative and intense, you'll get a different set of changes. We change based on our life experiences. This makes the "fixed brain" myth dead in the water and simply outdated and incorrect science. For example, we know that the human brain can and does grow new brain cells. Just as important, many of them survive, become functional, and best of all, we have something to do with that process (Eriksson et al., 1998).

This is pretty exciting, but there's more. We now know that exposure to domestic violence can, unfortunately, hurt a child's intelligence (Koenen, Moffitt, Caspi, Taylor, & Purcell, 2003).

Our brains change by the choices we make. Do we watch television or learn to play an instrument? We know that learning a skill such as playing an instrument or even driving a taxi can cause increase in brain structures (Gaser & Schlaug, 2003; Maguire et al., 2003).

There are other types of changes besides increases or decreases in brain mass. Researchers found that learning to master new learning, even playing a video game, will change blood flow and activity in the brain (Haier et al., 1992).

What does school do to the brain? We know that the more we study, the greater the changes in our brain! We also know that when students study hard, their brain actually increases in mass compared to those who mostly loaf at school (Draganski et al., 2006).

What we used to think was fixed (genes) is now known to be receptive to the environment. Thus, gene expression is powerful enough to even influence what used to be sacred between identical twins, metabolism (Berezovskii, Zelenskaia, Serebrovskaia, Zverkova, & Il'chevich, 1986).

So far, we have seen mostly positive effects of changes in the brain. Being more realistic, it can go the other way. As one might expect, negative influences such as drug abuse can alter brain structures, including our neurons (Farber & Olney, 2003).

What's the sum total of all this? Compared to students who take easier classes, we know that the hard workers get a bonus; their brain is better. We know that taking harder, more complex classes alters our brain by increasing the length of the brain cells' extensions, the dendrites (Jacobs, Schall, & Scheibel, 1993).

While we don't have direct control over kids' lives, there are many opportunities to change and vary the brains of our students in a positive way. They might include

- Skills/exercise
- Nutritional suggestions
- Stress levels
- Safe environments
- Challenging, novel learning
- Rest/settling time
- Meaning/relevance
- Feedback/error correction
- Mood, affect, personal connections

When you read that list, it ought to get you excited! Your students (or your own children) have brains that can be improved through environmental input. Brains change, both for the better and the worse,

Now let's summarize. We have learned that the brain is changing all the time. Processes such as cell growth (neurogenesis), dendritic branching, cell death (apoptosis), chemical changes, and genes all contribute to the changes. We know that genes have not one but two functions. The more recent discovery is that genes are highly susceptible to environmental input. This contributes to a wide body of knowledge that suggests our brains are in a state of constant flux.

IMPLICATIONS FOR EDUCATORS

This is good news for educators. Our students have enormous opportunities for positive changes. Evidence suggests an enormous capacity for a wide range of change. The fact that we often don't see dramatic changes does not mean they are impossible or even unrealistic. It means that the environmental input often remains largely static, and without any dramatic changes, the status quo is protected and the child stays the same. Here is how to remain more open to change and support higher expectations.

- Go ahead and influence and reduce negative teacher chatter

  "The apple doesn't fall far from the tree" is another way of saying, "I don't expect him to do well, since his parents are not very bright." Be positive and talk about possibilities of change, not negatives.

- Bring in unity and support

  Get as many teachers as you can on the same page to optimize student performance. The better the synergy, the faster the improvement.

- Talk to the parents about their child's opportunities
- Encourage better diet, more exercise, and lowered stress
- Follow the rules for learning

These are listed in the upcoming pages. They will ensure you're doing the most you can. Best resource: *Enriching the Brain* (Jensen, 2006).

PRINCIPLE 2: THE PRINCIPLE OF VARIETY: ALL BRAINS ARE UNIQUE

As different as a fingerprint, your brain is also unique to any other on earth. Even the brains of identical twins are different. What makes us unique? The simple answer is contributions from both genes and our environment. We know, for example, that humans vary dramatically in our maturation rates. This suggests that we avoid any curriculum or assessments that expect all students at a grade level to be on the same page on the same day (or week). There is no scientific support for trying to get all students to perform at the same level, based on age or grade level (Thompson et al., 2000).

Certainly, a genetic basis does not by itself explain the wide variances of a human being. As an example of our genetic similarities, all humans share 99.5 percent of the exact same DNA. Social, cultural, and environmental factors also contribute to cognition and behavior, both directly and indirectly. Directly, we can observe a command to a child or stimulus-response learning event. But indirectly, many factors exert actions on the brain by feeding back upon it to modify the expression of genes and thus the function of nerve cells. Our brains "learn" not just new content in school but also learn to alter key life processes, which is known as gene expression. In this way, genes continue to play a part in our lives, not by what was inherited but by what has been "learned" by life. Thus "nurture" is eventually expressed as "nature." It is both our genes and our experiences that make us unique.

How does environment make us unique? There are a host of factors that are each part of a unique recipe that one student gets but another doesn't. The ingredients in the "variation recipe" are likely to include the presence or absence of the following:

Bad moods	Playing an instrument
Distress	Daily walks
Learning	Diabetes
Doing yoga	Gene expression
Trauma	Watching TV
Nutrition	Hands-on science
Exercise	Boredom
Medications	Sleep

Nearly any environmental input, especially to excess, will lead to brain variations. For example, chronic stress will change our brain (it accelerates aging) compared to more typical on-off stress (Epel et al., 2004).

It has been demonstrated that students with special needs have a brain that is structurally and procedurally very different from those considered to be more typical (Baker, Vernon, & Ho, 1991; Castellanos & Acosta, 2002).

In the same vein, there is considerable evidence of brain differences in those determined to be gifted. While the type of brain difference varies, what does not vary is that there is a difference (Alexander, O'Boyle, & Benbow, 1966; Bogolepova, 1994; Jausovec & Jausovec, 2004).

We've all heard of learning styles. There are many models that have illuminated the differences among students, including the Gregorac, 4-MAT, Meyers-Briggs personality inventory, and the visual, auditory, and kinesthetic model. But is there any brain research that validates a "learning style" or even "personality style"? Yes, there is. Some people *do* use their brain preferentially, and that can generate a personality and learning profile (Fox, Henderson, Marshall, Nichols, & Ghera, 2005).

IMPLICATIONS FOR EDUCATORS

Taken as a whole, the evidence suggests a wide variation in human brains, both physically and functionally. This understanding strengthens the position of those who encourage the differentiation model. This principle suggests we ought to avoid grade-level comparisons, gender comparisons, age, school, or district-by-district comparisons. The only thing that makes sense is comparing one student to himself or herself at a later time. Here is how to add more variety, with more ways to help reach students:

- Amount of task time

  "You may take up to seven minutes. If you finish early, you can . . ."

- Modality

  If you show it, let them discuss it; if you tell them, let them draw it or perform it.

- Social conditions

  Individual, partners, small groups, teams, whole class, and so on

- Content complexity

  "You may choose Challenge Level 1, 2, or 3. Tell me which one fits you the best."

- Resources available

  Work by yourself, use texts, the Web, cooperative groups, and so on

Suggested Resource: *Different Brains, Different Learners* (Jensen, 2000)

PRINCIPLE 3: THE PRINCIPLE OF DEVELOPMENTAL SENSITIVITY

Many educators are frustrated because they are being asked to teach subjects that are simply developmentally inappropriate. Other educators notice that the more traditional approaches are not working. How can brain research inform us about the students' brains, and what might we be able to do about it? Let's take a quick look at three critical periods.

Birth to Five

Here the human brain is highly vulnerable; nature wants it to essentially "download" culture so infants have a chance to figure out what the world is like. It's almost like one is making a copy of a CD of the world. This indiscriminate (children's frontal lobes cannot evaluate, delete, or reframe negative input) downloading means that nearly every experience forms part of the lasting structures and messages that will run children's brains. Their brains are an energy bonfire, consuming twice as much glucose at age four than they will as an adult (Bower, 1999; Chugani, 1998; Tansey, Tansey, & Tachiki, 1994).

This is a brain that's trying to figure out how to survive in the world, and it will take in any and all experiences, even if they are negative. For example, if a child is exposed to parental abuse, disharmony, and trauma, the child's brain is highly likely to download the stress of uncertainty and the fear of losing one or both parents. That early distress may become a lifelong disability (Bunge, Dudukovic, Thomason, Vaidya, & Gabrieli, 2002; Gunnar, 2000).

We know that poverty in America can create lifelong problems for the human brain. The examples are many, and the primary problems are not economic. They demonstrate how a lack of resources influence lower-economic children: there's a lack of access to medical care, poor nutrition, unsafe lives, and chronic stressors (Bolger, Patterson, Thompson, & Kupersmidt, 1995; Lewit, Terman, & Behrman, 1997).

Young Children (Ages 5–11)

This is the prime age for sensory motor development and social skill building. Children can be exceptionally good at sports such as soccer, gymnastics, martial arts, dance, and playing music. There's no time to waste; these children need physical play and socialization more than they need seatwork. This does not mean avoiding math, reading, and science. It means it's a great time to blend in the other needs of the growing brain too (Hirsch-Pasek, Eyer, & Golinkoff, 2003).

Tweens to Teens (Ages 11–18)

A good metaphor for these years is starting the engine of a race car with an unskilled driver. The teen brain itself is different, and the teen skill set is different from what the same individual had as a preteen. This has been the recent focus of so many neuroscientific investigators that I can't begin to share all the latest discoveries with you here. We'll focus on just a few of the critical ones.

Many areas of the brain are still under major construction during adolescence. In fact, the changes are as dramatic as those happening in an infant's brain. The parietal lobes undergo major changes from ages 12 to 17. Certain subareas may double or triple in size. The frontal lobes, a big chunk of "gray matter," are the last area to mature, undergoing dramatic changes. Gray matter (brain cells) thickens first (between ages 11 to 13) and later thins (reduces 7 percent to 10 percent) between the ages of 13 and 20. There's a growth spurt of gray matter in the teen brain. This is followed by massive "pruning," in which about 1 percent of gray matter is pared down each year during the teen years while the total volume of white matter ramps up. This process is thought to shape the brain's neural connections for adulthood, based on experience (Paus et al., 1999).

The differences are dramatic; all these changes mean that a teen's brain needs more sleep time to consolidate, organize, and store new learning (Carskadon, Wolfson, Acebo, Tzischinsky, & Seifer, 1998).

Another metaphor to consider is that teen brains resemble blueprints more than skyscrapers. Instead of thinking about a teenage mind as an empty house that needs furnishings, educators and parents would do better to understand it as the framing of a house that still needs walls, wiring, and a roof. Stop treating teenagers like adults; they're not. They have the highest accident rate in cars and the highest incidence of brain injury of any age group. Does that sound like a thoughtful, mature brain? Teens are in a developmental fog and often make decisions even a nine-year-old would call stupid. Their brains are on a trajectory that rarely lets them make mature decisions (Sowell, Trauner, Gamst, & Jernigan, 2002).

They have sound biological reasons for the following patterns:

• *Susceptibility.* Teens are particularly susceptible to the risky extremes of novelty. Novelty juices up their unstable systems with brain chemicals like dopamine and noradrenaline. They choose short-lasting, immediate rewards over larger, delayed rewards. Their undeveloped frontal lobes play a significant role in reckless behaviors (Steinberg, 2005).

• *Lack of planning.* Teens have trouble anticipating the consequences of their behavior because they rely on their immature frontal lobes. They don't see options very well. They get confused easily under stress and rarely plan more than one move ahead. This is partly due to immaturity of frontal lobes (Durston, Hulshoff-Pol, & Casey, 2001).

• *Emotional stew.* Emotions are essential to learning, and teens are still learning how to understand and manage emotions. They are poor at reading emotions and weak at selecting the right friends and getting their mind outside their own world of feelings (Larson & Verma, 1999).

• *Crowd morality.* Teenagers will climb the moral ladder only as their frontal lobes develop. They spend an average of 28 hours a week on screens (TV, video, computer, movies, etc.)—all unsupervised, most of it alone (Strasburger & Donnerstein, 2000). To balance this, they often seek friendly (even if it's negative) peer clustering. But they're more likely to engage in risky behaviors when they're in groups than alone.

• *Difficulty in self-regulation.* Teens face a huge risk of chemical imbalances for behavioral and personality disorders such as anxiety, depression, stress, eating disorders, and shifts in sleep habits. Teens are more vulnerable to all of these than adults and have few coping skills. Much of the day they spend in apathy or slumping in angst (Eldridge, Galea, McCoy, Wolfe, & Graham, 2003).

• *Risk taking.* Teens are extremely vulnerable to addiction, and compared to adults, they are less cognizant of the effects of drug abuse and their addictions are harder to break. They see drugs as harmless, for the most part, and tend to believe that they can survive anything (Bardo, 2004).

IMPLICATIONS FOR EDUCATORS

This principle suggests that we might reorganize *when* we do things to maximize the brain's capacity to learn them. For example, learning a new language or musical instrument should be a K–5 activity, rather than one delayed for the later years.

Studies suggest that as students reach the age of approximately 12 years (until about 22 years), the body's clock modulates. The desire to go to bed later and get up later at this time appears to be biological in nature, rather than a response to peer pressure or socialization. The last couple of hours of sleep are critical to schoolday attention. To maximize student alertness, learning, and memory, researchers suggest that K–5 students continue to start at the early time of 7:30 a.m. But for students from Grades 6 to 12, the morning start time ought to be closer to 9:00 a.m. to accommodate a teen's natural biological tendency to go to bed later and wake up later.

Birth to Five (Mediation)

With children under the age of five, remember that they are going to download any and all experiences, emotions, and culture. Ensure not just quality time with youngsters, but quantity of quality time to protect them from stress, poor nutrition, trauma, neglect, and confusion. This is the time to focus on love, emotional reciprocity, movement, and certainty.

Young Children (Ages 5–11)

Encourage more guided exploration and plenty of social skill training. For parents, this is a great chance (before they get "too cool" when they're older) to enrich a youngster's life with traveling, exploring nature, visiting museums, participating in plays, taking martial arts, playing soccer, 4-H, dance classes, and scouts. In the classroom, now is the time to teach about drug abuse, ethics, nutrition, and morality.

Tweens to Teens (Ages 11–18)

Manage the risks, stay highly involved in their lives, ask questions, and reduce opportunities for dangerous activities. Remember, their brains are *not* adult yet, and they will not make mature, measured decisions. To maximize the teenage brain, guide it carefully through this dangerous time with focus, love, and involvement. It's a good time for 4-H, Outward

Bound programs, international travel, and camp programs. Do not put them in risky situations and expect adult-level decision making. Instead, partner, guide, and share experiences. Be a mentor and firm guide, not their best friend. Provide opportunities to make managed risks (indoor rock climbing, Outward Bound, skate parks, etc.). Focus on their strengths; their self-esteem is weaker than they'll let you on to.

PRINCIPLE 4: THE PRINCIPLE OF INTERACTION: WE HAVE A "SOCIAL BRAIN"

For most of the twentieth century, studies on cognition and achievement were conducted on individuals. Yet, most of us function in multiple, sometimes overlapping social networks. We have family, friends, acquaintances, and peer groups. Each of these social contacts influences us, and in turn, we influence them. The "social brain" is the term used for our built-in need to relate to ourselves as part of a social group. To do that we need some emotional intelligence and social skills. Social cognition is the processing of information, which leads to the accurate processing of the dispositions and intentions of others.

It is quite plausible that it was the development of complex social hierarchies, not our intellect, that contributed to the rapid increase in the size of the human brain. Areas of the brain dedicated to social structure are extensive and have been identified as the anterior prefrontal lobe, anterior cingulate, frontal gyrus, amygdala, fusiform gyrus, and posterior temporal lobe. We now know that our everyday social experiences have a significant influence on our emotional, academic, and physical being (Champagne & Curley, 2005).

Social and environmental events *at one level* of an organism (molecular, DNA, cellular, nervous system, organs, immune, behavioral, social, etc.) can profoundly influence events *at other levels* (Cacioppo, Berntson, Sheridan, & McClintock, 2001). We cannot think of ourselves and our contacts as fragmented; they must be part of a larger integrated picture. Even the neuroanatomical imagining map of the social cognitive brain is widespread. In order to process social information, we use areas of the brain that are associated with cognition, including the prefrontal cortex. This suggests that social contact at school may have a much more widespread influence than researchers earlier thought.

Social status is correlated with levels of cortisol and levels of a common neurotransmitter, serotonin, which is highly implicated in attention, memory, mood, and neurogenesis. Evidence also suggests that increases in social support will decrease blood pressure in hypertensive subjects (Uchino, Cacioppo, & Kiecolt-Glaser, 1996). Healthy social contact improves immune activity, and social stress weakens immune systems (Padgett & Sheridan, 1999). Researchers found social isolation is *just as devastating* a risk factor as is smoking or high blood pressure (House, Landis, & Umberson, 1988). Early social stressors can lead to lasting changes in the stress response system (Meaney, Sapolsky, & McEwen, 1985).

This new understanding is quite powerful, so let's review it. Social experiences can

- Change genetic expression
- Alter blood pressure
- Improve cognition
- Influence immune activity
- Modulate attention and memory
- Change stress response levels
- Regulate ovulation
- Influence brain chemistry

Why is all this important? Since the classroom and the school are significant social experiences, the brains of students *will be altered* by those experiences. To ignore the social influence on student brains is irresponsible. It is more than ethically essential to learn about this; it is mandatory that we understand and take responsibility for the ways we are shaping the brains of our learning customers. We know, for example, that academic achievement is enhanced when social contact is positive (Guay, Boivin, & Hodges, 1999).

We also know that although boys and girls experience relatedness differently (girls to each other and boys to the teacher), this social glue enhances achievement (Furrer & Skinner, 2003).

We also know that the broader context, which includes both the social experiences and the environmental setting, can influence our achievement.

Years ago, a group of psychologists were alerted to an amazing phenomenon. Brazilian youngsters with no formal school were doing fast (and accurate) math as part of their business transactions as street vendors. This is a classic example of context-dependent intelligence. Typically, the daily use of math by these adolescent street vendors in Brazil is in the 98–99 percent accuracy range. But in a nearby classroom, their accuracy drops by half, even on tasks that require the exact same skills (Carraher, Carraher, & Schliemann, 1985).

This is why we talk about the influence of the environment and social contexts (Ceci & Roazzi, 1994).

IMPLICATIONS FOR EDUCATORS

- Gathering Information

First, we can do a better job in gathering information about students' social conditions. How much time do students want to spend alone? How much time in pairs and how much time in groups or teams? This is critical to the success of the emotional learner. Depending on the age of students, the methods could vary. In some cases, small group discussion can work. For other teachers, it works to use simple gathering methods like thumbs up or down, though that's simplistic except for the most basic of information. Certainly, educators can gather information at the door as students enter and by simply watching and listening for changes over a baseline. Once this information is gathered, teachers should know more about student preferences, although variety will always be a good strategy.

- School Partners

Do not let any student, at the primary or secondary level, feel alone at school. Every single student should have a student to look after them (mentor or peer counselor) and an adult who knows them (homeroom class teacher or counselor). It is easy for students to feel lost and have no one to talk to.

- Quick Social Grouping

Much of the essential social time can happen from informal groupings. Ask students to stand up, walk 10 steps, and find a partner. Once with a new partner, students can pair share or interview each other, test a hypothesis, or review prior learning. Students can switch from one group to another or jigsaw their learning. Use simple social greetings in class with "turn-tos." When appropriate, you say, "Turn to your neighbor and say, 'Good Morning'" or "Turn to your neighbor and say, 'Good job!'"

- Social Events

Students need structured social conditions for a portion of their day. These social events might be assemblies, teams, and partners part of their day, mixed with some individual time. Then we want part of it to be choice, where students can go with their strengths and choose to be in the mode they work at best. Some choice is good in the environment for many reasons. Choice and control over their environment produces more social and less aggressive behaviors.

- Formal Grouping

Research on cooperative learning suggests that it produces better learning when compared to students competing against each other individually. Teams can work well too. The difference between teams and cooperative learning is simple. Teams are for a specific project. Think of collegiate or professional sports. The goal of those teams is to win games, and when the season is over, the team is dissolved. Teams are specific, high-performance structures that have a meaningful group goal. Cooperative groups may exist for a week, a month, or even a year, but there does not have to be a "grand" goal in mind. Bottom line, social bonding structures like either of these are important and valuable.

- Teaching Social Skills

It's easy to say we need better social skills in our youth. But these skills have to be taught by teachers who make it a priority. Most elementary teachers invest *some* time in it. By middle and high school, teachers are spending far less time on social skills. But if you do focus on them, what happens to grades? In general, they tend to get better. Why? Less time is spent having to repeat what is said; discipline the students and the overall mood and affect is higher.

PRINCIPLE 5: THE PRINCIPLE OF CONNECTIVITY: THE BRAIN IS AN INTEGRATED "SYSTEM OF SYSTEMS"

Our brain is far more connected to itself than we ever imagined. The old way of thinking about the brain envisions a separateness of mind, body, and emotions. That means movement only at recess or in PE classes; it means emotions get expressed in the counseling office, and classrooms are for cognition. That idea is history. Renowned neuroscientist Antonio Damasio (1994) reminds us that "the body may constitute the indispensable frame of reference for . . . the mind" (p. xvi); in fact, "reduction in emotion may constitute an equally important source of irrational behavior" (p. 53). All human processes are a function of the complex interplay of mind, emotions, body, and spirit. Everything we put into and see emerging from our students, from the simplest to the most complex cognitive expression, is a product of the unique and dynamic brain state that each of is in at any moment. This includes all actions, thinking, speaking, literature, music, and art. This principle reminds us that there is a basis, an engine and platform, from which all behaviors emerge. It's our mind-body-emotions-brain systems, and we call that our state.

Many highly respected neuroscientists—including Joseph LeDoux of New York University, Candace Pert of Georgetown University Medical Center, Jerome Kagan of Harvard Univeristy, and Antonio Damasio and Hanna Damasio of the University of Iowa—have put mind-body-emotional states in the public's consciousness. In fact, the publication of *The Cognitive Neuroscience of Emotion* (Lane & Nadel, 2000) formalized this burgeoning field, and Heilman (2000) shows how chemistry influences our emotional states. Each of our emotional states serves a purpose, and the right ones will help us pay better attention, create meaning, and even help us forge better memory pathways. Emotions influence and regulate behaviors, and they help us organize the world around us. You can't get more connected and related to than that!

This new understanding suggests that the role of emotional states such as threat, distress, and stress are huge in the big picture. When students feel in a state of fear, there's a perception of threat. Our brain has three choices when confronted with overwhelming threat. We can fight, flight, or freeze. In nature, animals will freeze when confronted if (a) they perceive there is no escape or (b) they are unlikely to win a fight. It's no different in the class-room. Students who feel threatened will fight back if they feel they can get away with it. Or they might just sit there and take it while stewing about it. Generally, they don't feel they can escape. But make no mistake about it— if there's a threat, the student's brain is going in high gear. Recent studies suggest that, whether perceived or real, the threat of violence in the learn-ing environment can have a negative impact on cognition. In animal stud-ies, it's clear that threat impairs the hippocampus and derails new learning (Diamond, Park, Hemen, & Rose, 1999). School stress associated with vio-lence impacts test scores, absenteeism, tardiness, and attention span (Hoffman, 1996). In a study of 35 fourth graders and 39 fifth graders, Nettles, Mucherah, and Jones (2000) concluded that children's perceived exposure to violence negatively affects test scores.

Distress, which is either acute stress or chronic stress over time, is devastating to school-age kids. The distress reduces the number of new brain cells produced (Gould McEwen, Tanapat, Galea, & Fuchs, 1997) and is linked with mood disorders (Brown, Rush, & McEwen, 1999). Chronic stress also impairs a student's ability to sort out what's important and what's not (Gazzaniga, 1988).

As you can guess, the way students feel is pretty important. At the least, it's uncomfortable when we are upset or stressed. But when the emotional states become far more acute or chronic, we are getting into very serious territory. Poor states can lead to lowered grades, minor damage to brain structures, and even less neurogenesis (the production of new brain cells).

IMPLICATIONS FOR EDUCATORS

This suggests to us as educators that we ought to pay close attention to the emotional states of our students, especially noticing the troubling states of frustration, distress, anger, apathy, fear, and hatred. These states all have suboptimal effects on learning, and until students are in better states, the learning will suffer. Here are some ways to be more proactive in managing student states.

- Role Model

  Wear your positive feelings on your sleeve! Model the love of learning and show enthusiasm for your job. For example, bring something with great excitement to class. Build suspense, smile, tell a true emotional story, show off a new CD, read a book, or bring an animal. Get involved in community work, whether it's for a holiday, disaster relief, or ongoing service. Let students know what excites you. We've all heard of infectious enthusiasm; it works!

- Celebrations

  Smart schools have pep rallies, guest speakers, poetry readings, community service efforts, storytelling, debates, clubs, sports, and dramatic arts. Teachers use acknowledgments, parties, high fives, food, music, and fun. A celebration can show off student work in different ways. For example, when students are finished mind-mapping something, ask them to get up and show their poster-sized mind map to eight other pairs of students. The goal is to find at least two things they like about it. As they carry around their mind map, they point out things to students, and they learn from their classmates. Play some celebration music, and everyone has a good time. Ideally, celebrations will be made "institutional" so students celebrate without a teacher prompt every time.

- Greater Movement and Music

  You may have already used music, games, drama, or storytelling to engage emotions. Even excitement and fun can help us remember things better. Our body releases dopamine and norepinephrine during movement and fun activities. Human studies show that these amines enhance long-term memory when administered either before or after learning. Create some positive emotions! It's better to have students remember the positives from school than the negatives. Use more standing than sitting, more walking than standing, and more organized activities than walking.

- Increased Classroom Rituals

  A ritual is a brief, prearranged activity that solves a recurring classroom problem such as getting attention. Rituals in your class can instantly engage learners. Those rituals could include clapping patterns, cheers, chants, movements, or a song. Use these to announce arrival, departure, a celebration, and getting started on a project. Make the ritual fun and quick, and change it weekly to prevent boredom. Each time teams complete their tasks, they could give a team cheer. Or they could have a special cheer for each member upon arrival and another for the close of the day. Obviously, rituals should be age appropriate.

- Writing

  The use of journals, discussions, sharing, stories, and reflection about things, people, and issues engages students personally. If there is a disaster in the news, ask students to write or talk about it. Current events or personal dramas work well too. If appropriate, students can share their thoughts with neighbors or peer groups. Help students make personal connections to the work they do in class. For example, if students are writing journals, have them read the letters to the editor in a local newspaper and discuss or even critique them. Students can choose an issue they are passionate about and submit letters to be printed.

Many other strategies can activate emotions. They include the use of music, competition, or simulations. Emotions can even be engaged in setting goals. Ask students to explain *why* they want to reach the goals they set. You might say, "Write down three good reasons why reaching your goals is important to you." Then have the students share their responses with others. The reasons are the emotions behind the goals and the source of the energy to accomplish them.

PRINCIPLE 6: THE PRINCIPLE OF MEMORY MALLEABILITY

The old way of thinking about memories was that they are much like a photograph. After all, we often look at photos to activate or verify our memories. We used to believe that you either formed a memory or not; it simply lasted if you used it, or it decayed otherwise. There's a bit of truth to that statement, but the larger discovery is that our memories are malleable (Schacter, 2001). They are malleable because we store them in pieces, like what you'd see in a kaleidoscope. The "pieces" of a memory are the properties of it, which include the sights, the sounds, the people, the smells, the location, your health, the day of the week, time of the day and surrounding circumstances, and so on. There are literally dozens of properties of a memory that would have to be bound together to have a perfectly intact memory (Shannon & Buckner, 2004). But it doesn't usually happen that way. We just can't pay attention to everything, all the time, to encode accurate memories. As a result, when we go to retrieve a memory, the memory pieces are usually incomplete and often flat-out wrong. This happens every day in a classroom as well as in the rest of the world. Our memories are typically fragmented and at times inaccurate.

Memories are formed many ways, and different kinds of life experiences encode differently (Fuster, 1995). As a result, each has a different likelihood of being recalled. The two primary categories for memories are generally considered to be explicit and implicit, also known as declarative and nondeclarative. Each general type of memory has its own strengths and weaknesses, as well as specific locations in the brain (Schacter, 2001).

We said that there were multiple pathways for our memory. One of the keys to enhancing memory is to use more than one. You might allow students to hear it or read it, then draw it or act it out.

We'll begin with the more well-known area, explicit learning. Explicit learning may be either semantic (words and pictures) or more episodic (autobiographical and a personal rendition of the memory versus learning about it second- or thirdhand). These two pathways are commonly known as the "what" and "where" pathways. The "what" pathways are typically processing learning in the temporal lobes, and the "where" pathways are typically processing input in the parietal lobes. It's the "Where were you when . . . ?" pathway that reminds us of a particular context or location along with the content. Ask the content question, "What did you have for dinner last night?" and most people immediately ask themselves first,

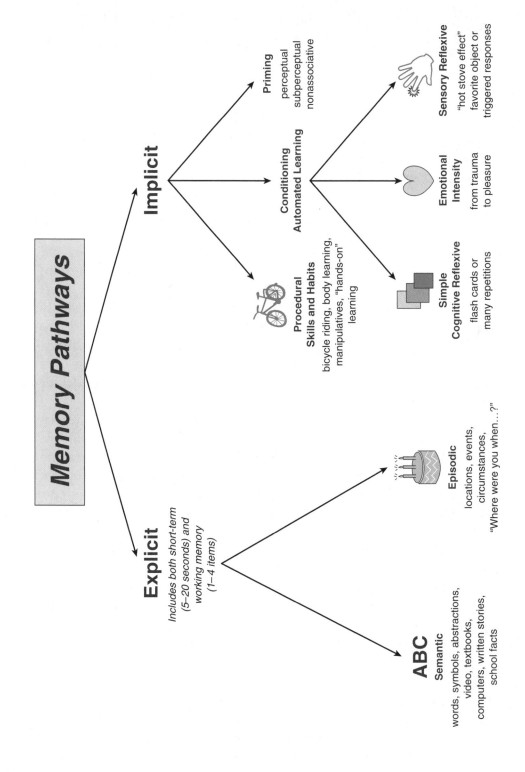

Memory Pathways

Explicit

Includes both short-term (5–20 seconds) and working memory (1–4 items)

ABC
Semantic

words, symbols, abstractions, video, textbooks, computers, written stories, school facts

Episodic

locations, events, circumstances, "Where were you when…?"

Implicit

Priming

perceptual
subperceptual
nonassociative

**Procedural
Skills and Habits**

bicycle riding, body learning, manipulatives, "hands-on" learning

**Conditioning
Automated Learning**

**Simple
Cognitive Reflexive**

flash cards or
many repetitions

**Emotional
Intensity**

from trauma
to pleasure

Sensory Reflexive

"hot stove effect"
favorite object or
triggered responses

"*Where* was I?" The *location and being there* triggers the content. A common example is "Where were you when 9/11 happened?"

The other major type of memory is implicit. Within that category are conditioned responses, reflexive, emotional, and procedural memories. These motor memories are often known as motor memory, body learning, or habit memory. It's expressed by student responses, actions, or behaviors. It's activated by physical movements, sports, dance, games, theater, and role play. Even if you haven't ridden a bike for years, you can usually do it again without practice. Procedural memory appears to have unlimited storage, requires minimal review, and needs little intrinsic motivation (Bailey, Kandel, & Si, 2004).

What we learn can begin as explicit (taught to us), yet later become reflexive. This memory pathway can be subdivided into emotional memories (favorite song from high school, first kiss, a car accident, etc.) and nonemotional associative memories (I say hot, you say cold; I say up, you say down; I say in, you say out). I reach my hand out to shake your hand, and your hand reaches out without a thought. There are only two ways that new learning can become reflexive: either intense sensory input (trauma, celebrations, etc.) or repetition. The importance of understanding that there are multiple pathways is simple: more pathways mean stronger memories.

IMPLICATIONS FOR EDUCATORS

This suggests to us as educators that we make memory encoding, revising, and updating a priority. But some of our memories are implicit. That means we may know it but might not know that we know it. Surprisingly, a great deal of what we learn and what we know is not taught to us. It is simply "picked up." The process of acquisition allows for vast amounts of material to influence us through our senses. This suggests you allow the environment to do some of the teaching through posters, examples, role modeling, and other students' work. Never assume that because your students don't recall information easily, they don't know it. It may be stored in a different pathway. Try alternative ways to discover if they know it. Here are some ways to strengthen our malleable memories.

- How We Retrieve Our Memories

  For maximum recall, do error correction, then store learning in multiple pathways. Then ensure the learner repeats the learning two to four times within the first hour. Review again the next day and again within a week and a month to solidify the memory.

- Semantic Learning (words, text, lecture, pictures)

  Teach students how to make and use acronyms, key words, peg words, word associations, and mnemonics. Remind them that all reading must be processed as it's read by mapping, journaling, or discussion. Encourage students to create multiple categories and groupings for their learning. Ask students to draw it out or make a flowchart or pictogram.

- Episodic

  Allow students to learn standing up, sitting on the floor, or sitting on the desk. Prepare lessons that take the class outside, in the cafeteria, or on a field trip. Bring in guest speakers, change the lighting, let kids wear costumes, and so on. Remember the movie *Dead Poet's Society*? Experiences that engage your students' imaginations and emotions and are novel in character and location will be ascribed a special memory address in the brain that will be easier to recall.

- Procedural

  Ensure that students get to move as a way to embed learning. Provide motion, hands-on learning, manipulatives, stretch breaks, drama, theater, and role play.

- Reflexive

  Students can learn through the productive engagement of strong emotions as well as with flash card-type learning that becomes automated with multiple repetitions.

- Enhance Working Memory

  Students will remember very little past a few seconds of input. Strengthen the short-term or temporary memory; it allows us to hold a small number of things in our head for a short time period. This is an absolutely essential capacity for students to have in order to keep up in class. You can strengthen working memory several ways. First, practice in memory skills does work wonders. Even world-renowned memory experts practice to enhance their working memory capacity. Second, teach students memory devices such as acronyms and mnemonics. Finally, enhance dopamine levels. Dopamine supports working memory. You can do this though quick successes like a fast review, celebrations, or even some rapid gross motor activity like walking around the room (Denenberg, Kim, & Palmiter, 2004; Tanaka, 2002).

- Reality Checks

  It's not likely any student is going to remember a page of written text, much less a few sentences. When you ask students to read a chapter, insist that they stop after each page and take some notes. If it's in a classroom, use a variety of activities that engage partners such as having one of the partners read and having the other map out the content. If you're lecturing, after just a few short minutes, let them pair up and reteach. If they struggle, add another activity in a larger group to do error correction and consolidation, such as a group discussion with a prompting handout.

- Use Varieties of Repetition

Build up strong representations of the learning over time. Avoid hoping for a quick one-time success. Use priming and preexposure by giving vocabulary words days and weeks in advance. Use graphics, illustrations, and models that you post up for maximum clarity in learning complex subjects. Use daily reviews with partners or teams to get feedback on prior learning as well as revise any misconceptions.

PRINCIPLE 7: THE PRINCIPLE OF RESOURCE CONSUMPTION

Dealing with emotional, social, and home stressors consumes resources that could be used for learning.

Learning Requires *Physical* Resources

Help your learners understand the relationship between nutrition and learning and memory. Studies confirm that a definite measurable relationship exists between what one eats and how one feels and performs. Reacting to the foods we eat, dopamine and norepinephrine are the alertness chemicals. Serotonin is the calming chemical. Protein eaten alone or before a carbohydrate increases "alert brain power." On the other hand, carbohydrates eaten without protein will result in an increased sense of relaxation.

There are many ways to influence the eating behaviors of kids. Talk to them about how to fix better breakfasts and pack smarter lunches. Speak about nutrition at open houses. Give parents nutritional guidelines. Role-model good eating habits. Put healthier foods in school vending machines. Work with the food service staff to prepare more nutritious meals. The human brain is 78 percent water. When dehydration occurs, attention, critical thinking, learning, and memory are impaired. Allow water bottles in your classroom or remind students to at least drink water before class to avoid dehydration.

Of those who *bring a lunch* to school, four out of five get poor nutrition; their lunches fail to meet the USDA government guidelines for both quality and proportions of grains, proteins, fats, carbohydrates, oils, and sugars (Lino, Basiotis, Gerrior, & Carlson, 2002). Those who *buy at school* don't do much better (Wildey et al., 2000). Overall, it's not easy to eat right for learning. Proper nutrition also includes sufficient protein, trace minerals, liquids, and B vitamins. We learn best with less carbohydrates and a nibbling diet. Ensure your learners have the critical nutrients for good learning and memory. This includes sufficient hydration, glucose, multiple vitamin and mineral supplements, and a low transfat diet. In general, proteins are more of an upper for the brain, complex carbohydrates supply long-term energy, and dark vegetables have antioxidant effects. Get enough vitamins A, B, and E, because each has been shown to influence memory and recall (Bellisle, 2004; Kennedy & Scholey, 2000; Maughan, 2003).

Practical Suggestions

Talk to parents about nutrition

Role-model good nutrition

Provide clear facts and alternatives to junk foods

Bring in articles on better eating

Direct students to movies/DVDs (e.g., *Fast Food Nation*)

Emotional Readiness Is Key

Students are at their best at learning when they have feelings of safety, are vested in the learning, experience low to moderate stress, can choose relevant, novel learning, and have feelings of optimal challenge. Students also do better with a goal orientation and the knowledge and confidence that they have sufficient assets to make the learning happen. All these are emotional qualities. Anxiety in students consistently diminishes their processing skills (Mogg, Bradley, & Hallowell, 1994). We simply do worse under moderate to significant threat because strong emotions impair cognitive processing (Simpson, Snyder, Gusnard, & Raichle, 2001). Classrooms that allow threats, bullying, harassment, and put-downs impair student learning (Wessler, 2004).

There are many, many ways to get kids vested in the learning process. Some teachers help build student strengths, so they're more confident. Others build relationships and trust. And other teachers use good old-fashioned curiosity.

——————— CASE STUDY ———————

Mrs. Jefferson's Class

Mrs. Jefferson's memory was that years ago, her third graders loved to read. Today, it seems they're more interested in video games than reading. She has tried to motivate them by using choice and allowing students to write and then read their writing in class. But she still had problems getting them more emotionally vested. Then she came up with an idea. A crazy one, but it was worth trying.

She pulled out one of her favorite books for third graders, The Hidden Stairs and the Magic Carpet *by Tony Abbott (1999). The plot revolves around a character named Eric (what a coincidence) who discovers, with Julie and Neal, a magic staircase to another world. Mrs. Jefferson preread the story and identified several places where there's a natural cliff-hanger spot. It leaves readers hanging in the air so they feel compelled to get to the next sentence.*

When Mrs. Jefferson got to the first cliff-hanger spot, she stopped and paused. She asked the students, "Where might the story go from here? Could someone get lost or hurt? Who?" The questions really stimulated the students' appetite for more. But of course, there was no more. Now it was the students' turn. To find out what happened, they had to go read the rest themselves.

The first time she did this, her strategy reached a few students, but after Mrs. Jefferson started learning how to create even more mouth-watering suspense, more and more students got more into reading. The process became fun for Mrs. Jefferson too.

———————————— ● ● ● ————————————

Practical Suggestions

Show enthusiasm and caring

Allow time for stretching at the start

Make the classroom safe—no put-downs/no bullying

Use goal setting (choice is good) and planning

Link the content with personal connections

Set aside time for journaling and sharing

Stair-step the process, starting small

Organize student feedback (specific, prompt, task, and local)

Create small group discussions with group leaders

Imbue content with huge relevance or meaning

Invest in student asset building like study skills and memory tools

Input Limitations

The younger we are, the more our brain downloads from the environment with reckless abandon. The older we get, the more it seems we slow down new learning to preserve existing learning. Many brain structures and processes actually serve to limit the quantity of new information getting to the brain. They include our limited attention span, lack of coherence, and weak learner background (McNamara, 2001). In addition, our brain needs time for constant nutrients to support the protein recycling needed for memory (Frank & Greenberg, 1994). Other processes that can slow down new content acquisition include working memory (Cowan, 2001), limited glucose supplies, hippocampus processing delays, insufficient sleep time (Wesseling & Lo, 2002), synaptic formation and adhesion time (Goda & Davis, 2003), and later memory consolidation (Wiltgen, Brown, Talton, & Silva, 2004).

Much other evidence supports significant limitations on what students can hold in their heads (Callicott et al., 1999; Klingberg, 2000; Lachter & Hayhoe, 1995). This is mental juggling known as the cognitive load theory. Research suggests we be cautious with the rate of delivery of instructional information (Carlson, Chandler, & Sweller, 2003). All the evidence points to the conclusion that we do better when there's learning followed by processing and a pause (Bower, 1987; Colicos & Goda, 2001). Many teachers have learned this key understanding from my workshops. One of them was Barbara Mercer at the Vancouver School for the Arts & Academics in Vancouver, Washington. She has classes of sixth- to twelfth-grade kids who are pulled out for special one-on-one services with a tutor because they are struggling. Before they go back into their regular ed classes, they are "skilled up" to ensure they can keep up with the pace and content.

———————— CASE STUDY ————————

Brain-Compatible Learning in Action

We (my teaching partner Mike Brasch and I) have focused on threat reduction with students who are very low readers by engaging them with lots of self-assessment, personal connections, personal stories, humor breaks, music for transition, better mental states, having enough water and movement for every-one's brain food, stretching to start each class, and lots of partner and small group work. My kids understand exactly how their brains work, and they know why they need settling time (to allow for better connections) after every 20 minutes of input. They even share the fact that they have to ask their other teachers for settling time to make better connections! Pruning during sleep is something they come into class discussing and are very anxious for a quick "brain check" of the previous day's information to see what if anything was pruned. The role of the hippocampus is very clear to them, and they laugh about the fact that their brain's "media specialist" is hard at work looking for the information that it stored the previous night. We have lots of fun with all of this cool brain information, but meanwhile our data are showing huge gains in literacy skills as we go along through this year.

———————————— ● ● ● ————————————

Your low background learners must have high coherent texts or they'll do poorly (McNamara, 2001). This suggests you might want to test out your text on selected students to ensure it serves their needs well.

Practical Suggestions

Use more spiraling, previewing, doubling back, and reviewing strategy.

Pause more often. Give extra wait and think time for processing.

Chunk information into bite-sized bits.

Use daytime power naps, which are good, as are brief closed-eye breaks.

Do more advance organizing and previewing.

NECESSITY FOR PROCESSING

The value of greater elaboration in the learning processing can be seen through a simple experiment. Lecture to adults for 8–10 minutes. Then ask them to stand, find a partner, and share what they've learned from the lecture. The majority of the adults will find it difficult to talk past 30–45 seconds, meaning that they're at less than 10 percent absorption of the spoken content. With younger students, the numbers are even more discouraging. Your novice learners will create very weak, shallow representations based on initial rough drafts in their minds. As these concepts migrate from working memory to their hippocampus, they will have developed sketchy patterns and sometimes even mental models (Johnson-Laird, 1980) based primarily on a pinball game style selection of features. Without time for more elaborate processing, your learners, especially your novice learners, will have discouragingly inaccurate understandings of the content. It will take strong work to get closer to accurate models (Levin, 1988).

CASE STUDY

Mr. Bernstein

After sorting through the latest round of student quizzes, Mr. Bernstein had an uneasy thought. His students seemed to be grasping his eleventh-grade curriculum at a superficial level. His world history class seemed to be enjoying the material, but they didn't know much more than what a fifth or sixth grader would know. Typically, Mr. Bernstein would lecture and have the students write a paper from their class notes. He decided that he needed to lecture less and allow them to do some digging into the subject matter differently. His new plan had two parts to it.

The first part was teaching students how to analyze the content differently. He found some case studies to use with his class, but he needed more. He worked with his students to develop specialized rubrics to analyze the case studies from many angles. In fact, sometimes the students had to get more information from the Internet to complete the rubric. This got the students to think about the material in different ways.

The second part of his plan was to have the students contribute six questions. Three of them would be summary type, and three of them would be more detail oriented. On the very next weekly quiz, Mr. Bernstein noticed some changes. First, the students looked forward to the quiz to see if Mr. Bernstein had used their questions. Second, the students actually did a bit better.

———————————— ● ● ● ————————————

Fortunately, with your more expert learners (often few and far between), the picture is better. Instead of forming sketchy representations based on often irrelevant features (size of text, color, quirky shapes, length of material, catchy words, etc.), your experts will develop stronger mental models based on underlying, often fundamental principles (the how, the why, cause and effect, etc.). This more sophisticated understanding will serve the students much better, but it didn't come easy (Chi, Feltovich, & Glaser, 1981). This learner usually started along the same path as the novice, and at one time also focused on features. In either case, both learners will have either fundamental or peripheral flaws in their understanding. Even starting very young, the elaboration and error correction strategies can have a significant, positive impact on learning (Willoughby, Porter, Belsito, & Yearsley, 1999).

Processing for Accuracy

Make the assumption that your learners will *not* get complex learning the first time. The trial and error process allows students to move quickly from flawed understanding and mental models to more accurate representations. Generally, feedback is better if it's given more rather than less often, but overdoing it can hurt performance (Schroth, 1997). Feedback is better (Goodman, Wood, & Hendrickx, 2004) when it's built into the task; that is, the results of the task itself provide corrective insights (Kluger & DeNisi, 1996; Latham, 1997).

Feedback and error correction is essential, and meaning making is automatic (but it may not be the meaning you were hoping for). As an example, some students may decide that learning about the ancient Greeks is a big waste of time. In this case, the teacher would see that she failed to frame the learning or make it relevant from the start.

Suggestions From the Research on Feedback

- Ensure mixing some negative feedback with mostly positive (35–65 percent)
- Direct feedback at specifics, not global (say, "You were five minutes late," instead of "You're lazy and unreliable")
- Provide a variety of formats (writing, verbally, peer, Web, etc.)
- Limit at the onset of the task, increasing as learner gains mastery
- Avoid using competition or comparison as feedback ("Your class ranking is moving up!")
- Focus feedback on the task and keep it limited to local and specific suggestions ("Put the AB function on the left side of the equation, not right")

This means you can help students stay motivated by finding ways to give their learning sufficient error correction. We've all heard that feedback is the breakfast of champions. There's some truth to it; feedback is a primary driver in student motivation. The secret is learning to get the quantity and quality of feedback directly to your students. How can you do it? First, don't try to do it all yourself. Use feedback-driven activities that can do it for you. These include the following:

- Peer editing
- Think, pair, share, and get feedback
- Audio/video and debrief
- Model building, trying its functionality, comparing it to another
- Mentor feedback
- Rubrics for evaluation
- Real-world results—what happened?
- Cooperative learning
- Simulations to test a hypothesis
- Galleries walk with feedback
- Student presentations with audience feedback
- Games with competition
- Mirrors to watch, reflect, and discuss
- Author's chair or fishbowl processes
- Checklists to measure results
- Hypothesis building and trying it out, then debrief

Processing for Meaning

The brain is generally poor at learning random data and isolated facts. It constantly seeks to make sense out of what is happening. Your students don't really want information; they want meaning. The search to make meaning out of our lives seems to be innate. Until *you* understand what makes meaning, you can't help *them* get it. We gain meaning three ways: patterns, emotions, and relevance. We learn best with context, the big picture, real-life learning, and interdisciplinary relationships. When things are emotional, they are assigned more meaning too. As a rule, our brain naturally seeks meaning. As learning catalysts, we can either impede or facilitate that process. The primary variables are as follows:

Framing. This is the "why" that surrounds the learning of anything. Studying for a test can become framed as "Passing this test is how you'll get into college."

Relevance. Connect information with other known, relevant, or valuable information. Use associations with prior knowledge to make it meaningful. For example, "This city is where your mother was born. Let's see what we can learn about how she grew up."

Emotion. Emotional experiences "code" our learning as important, whether it is or is not important. Emotions can be on a scale from low to high valence (boring to intense). They may also be rated as more negative to highly positive.

Context/Patterns. Information in isolation has little meaning. Each puzzle piece is always part of something larger. Meaning comes from understanding the larger pattern. Some examples include community service work, neighborhood issues, health, romance, eliciting past experiences, and complex real-life projects.

Environment Matters

Do you have a heater or air conditioner in your house? Do you vacation in your own house or try to get away? How important is water to a fish? These questions are asked to elicit a response about how you value your home and work environment. Chances are, your environment means a great deal to you. Our brain is highly responsive to environments that may trigger stress responses, alertness, lethargy, or hormones. When a consulting group studied the effects on school environment on 8,000 students, the result was startling (Heschong Mahone Group, 2003). The following were found to have a statistically significant (greater than 5 percent) effect on student achievement:

Amount of bright lighting available

Operable windows

Direction the classroom windows faced

New or old (and noisy) fluorescent bulbs

Amount of glare in the classroom

Temperature in class

While it's difficult to quantify the overall effect of environment on learning, several have found a profound influence (Moore & Lackney, 1993; Schneider, 2002). At the low end, estimates place the effects of school environment on student success as low as 1–3 percent, yet it may well be as high as 40–50 percent or more at the upper end.

Practical Suggestions

Maintain a constant, adequate level of bright lighting (at least 2,000 lux) in your classroom. Bright lighting helps reduce drowsiness in class by suppressing the production of melatonin in the brain.

Get an acoustic analysis of your classrooms. Many may need some kind of wall buffers. Others may need to be fitted for sound systems with teachers on a Wi-Fi setup with wireless microphones for mobility.

Limit student exposure to darkened lecture halls and similar environments for extended periods. When such exposure is necessary, include low-level background lighting (from a hallway or a window).

Give teachers the ability to regulate the classroom temperature with either a thermostat, fans, curtains, blinds, doors, or a skylight.

During periods of limited sunlight in the fall and winter, encourage learners to get proper exercise. Take them on frequent field trips and brisk walks, and hold PE classes outdoors when possible, rather than in a gym. Incorporate ample movement in the classroom as well.

Minimize the distractions outside the windows. Add a row of plants or have students face another direction.

During periods of decreased sunshine in October through March, make sure students are exposed to as much natural sunlight as possible; open classroom blinds and skylights.

Settling Time

Our brain is not designed for continuous input. In fact, ideally, we would learn, process it, and go for a walk or take a nap. Just getting our attention and keeping it is quite a challenge—unless you're putting survival at risk. Then you get our attention *real* fast. Interestingly, our brain is designed for ups and downs, not constant attention. The old notion of teachers getting students' attention and keeping it is outdated. Having perfect attention from a class is not only statistically improbable but it's bad for learning. Why? Downtime allows our brain to "fix" neural connections, leading to better memory. Downtime allows a learner to construct meaning out of an experience. Much of our learning, which is done on a nonconscious level, without reflection, remains on that level. You can either have your learners' attention, or they can be making meaning for themselves, but not both at the same time.

Our body clocks seem to run in 90- to 110-minute cycles. These low-to-high energy or relaxation-to-tension cycles are called ultradian patterns. These shifts affect our academic performance (Gordon, Stoffer, & Lee, 1995). They are affected by shifts in our breathing and energy levels and dramatically affect our learning and perception of ourselves. Generally speaking, learners will focus better in the late morning and early evening, and they tend to be more pessimistic in middle to late afternoon. Physical activity or emotional engagement can modify the brain's normal rhythm. A break that incorporates physical exercise is an excellent way to alter a low cycle.

Here's the mind-body connection. Your body has high-low cycles of about 90–110 minutes. When students are at the top of these cycles, they're much more attentive. At the bottom of the cycle, energy drops, and attention and learning do too. Learn to ride with the cycles and you'll have fewer problems. When your students' energy is low, either do quiet reflective activities or plan on adding movement, or you'll get groggy learners. Learn to give physical breaks that are super brain energizers, and you'll keep energy up too.

Practical Suggestions

Shorten required attention time

Have students stay busy with more class jobs

Increase choice in learning

Take the time for a quick stretch or dance time

Boost relevance, choice, and engagement

Utilize more nonconscious learning (posters, people, music, projects)

Provide a variety of learning experiences that engage more senses

Use cross laterals to wake up the brain

Slowing Down for a Rest

Our resource-hungry brain uses the quiet time to build synaptic connections, consolidate learning, and eventually transfer short-term to long-term memories. Axons from the projecting neuron create an electrochemical signal to the receiving surface of the neighboring dendrite. The junction area is known as the synapse. Initially, the synapse is highly unstable, right at the beginning of new learning. A variety of factors stabilize this connection to ensure that the memory is accurate and fixed. There are extensions from the axons known as boutons and spines from the dendrites, which form the connections. There also may be neuromodulators like cortisol or norepinephrine that accelerate or enhance the potential memory. A significant limitation is the rate at which the brain can recycle the necessary chemicals, particularly proteins required in memory formation (Wesseling & Lo, 2002).

Different types of learning require a different amount of time to stabilize. Surprisingly, the amount of time needed to connect, stabilize, and strengthen a memory ranges from several minutes (not seconds) to several hours (Dudai, 2004). Just to record and remember *where* things are, our hippocampal neurons require five to six minutes of experience to form stable spatial representations (Frank, Stanley, & Brown, 2004). Typically, it takes between 15 and 60 minutes for the synapse to form and become stable for most explicit learning. The majority of presynaptic boutons are stable in efficacy and position over a period of 90 minutes (Hopf, Waters, Mehta, & Smith, 2002). Most complex implicit learning, primarily skill learning, requires up to six hours of settling time to solidify (Shadmehr & Holcomb, 1997). Synapses stay intact partly through synaptic adhesion, a process that binds the connecting axon and dendrite together. It is not known at this time whether different learning in different areas of the brain would constitute "competing" stimuli. But it is clear that too much information constitutes an overload similar to rewriting a CD with new information after it's full of old information.

The third area of the brain that limits our new explicit learning is the hippocampus. It seems that nature is more conservative with our existing information and prevents content overload from new learning. If the learning is not emotional or relevant and not heard from again, the hippocampus might not even encode it. But if the new learning is repeated over time, even just an hour, it's got a better chance of being remembered (Colicos, Collins, Sailor, & Goda, 2001). New information may travel the route of working memory to our hippocampus and await further information regarding saliency. Our hippocampus becomes our temporary holding and organizing area for all new explicit learning. It looks much like two small,

C-shaped structures, each buried in the temporal lobes, one on each side of the brain. Sometimes our hippocampus holds information for hours, sometimes for weeks, before letting it go or distributing it to the rest of the cortex for long-term memory (Wiltgen, Brown, Tatton, & Silva, 2004). The hippocampus does not have unlimited storage space. It learns fast, but it's more like a flash memory stick than a huge hard drive. In fact, its role in the brain is more like a surge protector than a library. Overload the hippocampus and very little gets learned.

Practical Suggestions

Space out the learning. Instead of shorter, more defined units, use a more spiraling, previewing, and reviewing strategy (Bower, 1987).

Pause more often when presenting new material. Once every 30–60 seconds allows the brain time to better assimilate new information (Di Vesta & Smith, 1979).

Allow more wait time and more think time for processing (Stahl, 1994).

Have daytime naps. They're good! (Mednick et al., 2002; Mednick, Nakayama, & Stickgold, 2003). If that's impossible researchers suggest that a brief closed-eye break can do miracles (Maquet, Peigneux, Laureys, & Smith, 2002).

Prepare the learners better with both content and process priming.

Use continual reviews to strengthen existing learning.

Provide mini breaks for stretching, reflection, or movement.

Give half-filled-in notes that provide key words to remember.

Use enough variety in your teaching so students rarely recognize that they're constantly transforming the learning into different understandings.

Repetition and Revision

The human brain works, as you've no doubt heard, on the principle that more use and more repetition is better for enhancing the memory. Somewhere, somehow, someone started the theory that if it's brain-based learning, repetition is bad for the brain. That's baloney. The bottom line is that repetition strengthens connections in the brain. But the repetition has to be accurate too.

───── CASE STUDY ─────

Postviewing With Lori Brickley

Ms. Brickley is a former teacher of the year in her Poway, California, district and is so good, I'd pay to watch her teach. On this visit I had brought some educator friends from Hong Kong with me, and we all sat quietly in the back of her biology class. The lesson was cycling back over previously learned material. The students were enjoying the fact that they obviously knew their material. Soon, I could see why her students were so comfortable and confident with the material.

About halfway into the class, she brought out a huge pile of folksy placards for a quick postview. Some had sentences with blanks to fill in, others simply had key words or pictures. In a playful, rhythmic, and clearly purposeful way, she held up each placard, repeated the phrase, or described the picture. Then she waited for the class to do their part. Sometimes it was word association, other times it was a fill-in. At first, responses were hesitant, given the intrusion of international visitors.

But in time, all seemed to jump in. Over and over, immediate repetition of key words and key concepts made more sense, even to the visitor. It's simple, but with enthusiasm and novelty, she made the process work. Her students have strong achievement scores for a reason. Repetition builds confidence and the background for the deeper levels of mastery. Students feel smarter, and they take that confidence to test time.

───── ● ● ● ─────

Remember, it's the repetition that tells our brain "It's worth saving—keep this!" In fact (remember this), recent research suggests *it takes up to four repetitions for our brain to remember most things* (Goda & Davis, 2003).

That turns your brain from a tangled jungle of neurons into sizzling intellect, or at least one with a decent memory. There is nothing brain antagonistic about repetition—we've all heard that "Neurons that fire together, wire together." When neural connections are stimulated repeatedly, and we pay attention, they strengthen significantly (Kilgard & Merzenich, 1998). Bad repetition occurs only when it's too boring. The single greatest difference between novel learners and expert learners is the quantity of time spent practicing (Ericsson, 1996). There's no way around it; repetition is good for many reasons:

- It can overcome the difficulties associated with low-background students.
- Existing memories are unstable—repetition can stabilize and strengthen them.
- Many students don't think content's important—until it's repeated often, so this triggers the need to learn.
- Often the learner does not get it right the first time—repetition supports accuracy.
- Increased repetition can also increase learner confidence.
- Our brain becomes less energy hungry and far more efficient when we need to do the same task again.

Practical Suggestions

Have students create a written quiz. Variations include (a) each small group contributes three to five questions for a larger quiz, (b) each small group creates quiz of 15 questions to trade with another small group, or (c) every student contributes two questions to the whole group.

Ask students to summarize the learning in a paragraph and then pair share.

Have students create a graphic organizer. Variations include (a) students working on their own, (b) students working with a partner on a flip chart paper, or (c) students doing a mind map and passing it around for others to add to it.

Ask students in groups of three to four to summarize a key point in a rhyming one-liner review. Have them add a little choreography and present it to the class.

PART III

So What;
Now What?

ASKING BIG QUESTIONS: WHAT'S IN A BRAIN-COMPATIBLE CURRICULUM?

- Developmentally Appropriate Lesson Plans and Strategies

Many students are currently being asked to do things too early for their age. As an example, in the countries with the highest literacy in the world (New Zealand and Denmark), students are not expected to read until one to three years later than in the United States.

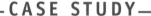 CASE STUDY

A Struggling Student

Alejandro was a likable first grader. From Day 1, the teacher and other students seemed attracted to his smile, his energy. But soon after, it became clear that he was struggling. In small cooperative groups, he seemed out of sorts and didn't contribute. Soon other students began to shy away from him. A cascade effect seemed to take place where his participation dropped in the full classroom too. Alejandro seemed a bit shell-shocked by all the business of school and the constant changes and demands of attention. His teacher, Ms. Templeton, had some ideas. After a meeting with Alejandro, his parents, and the school counselor, separately, then together, the data gathering was complete. The thinking was that one of three choices might help.

One was to hold back Alejandro a year until he was more mature. This might give him a better chance to succeed and prevent any permanent effects from the stress. Another choice was to refer him to another nearby school with smaller classes. Sometimes this gives students enough attention and reduces the pressure to perform.

In this case, there was another teacher, Ms. Suarez, at the same school who already had a smaller class and had some experience with younger students. She put no pressure on Alejandro to read and instead focused on love of words, vocabulary, and interesting stories. Once he was in the new class, his confidence seemed to return. Within another 12 months, Alejandro was reading.

———————————— ● ● ● ————————————

- Culturally Appropriate Curriculum (general and specific)

  Many classes are not taught with the culture of the students in mind. For example, Hispanics comprise over 20 percent of the population at large, but we rarely ask questions of what is appropriate in the Hispanic culture.

- Integrated and Interdisciplinary Material

  Much of what is taught is far too compartmentalized. Many units could be taught simultaneously, in several subjects, to increase interest.

- Lessons Relevant to Students and Teacher

  Many students sit through classes, particularly at the secondary level, that have little relevance to the real world. Only the vocational education classes do well in this area.

- Awareness of Gender Differences

  The idea, based on how genders interact, would include (a) mixed sex at the primary level, (b) same sex in all core academic classes at secondary level, and (c) mixed sex in all electives.

- Social and Emotional Literacy

  These are core life skills and should be taught at every grade level. Put special emphasis on quality social skills. These are the skills that build relationships, smooth over friction, and even help get jobs.

- Nutritional and Health Information

  This influences health, weight, cognition, memory, and mood. All students should understand what's in foods and what they do to our brain and body. Be sure to give students necessary drug and toxin awareness.

- Early Music, Dance, and Arts Training

  There is a wide body of evidence that early arts training strengthens the biological, emotional, social, and cognitive development of humans. This should be at least 10 percent of all curriculums.

- Learning-to-Learn Skills

  Never assume that students actually know how to (a) prioritize, (b) study, (c) memorize, (d) take notes, (e) be organized, or (f) a host of other skills. If you don't teach them, who will?

- Daily Physical Activity

  There is significant and overwhelming evidence of the positive value of daily physical activity. It reduces stress, builds cognition, improves flexibility, stabilizes brain chemicals (mood), and even helps us grow more brain cells. If you reduce it, your test scores will flatten out.

All of these curriculum concepts can be made safe to use by the administrator and can be made relevant through the skills of the teacher and the students' own initiative.

BRAIN-COMPATIBLE TEST-TAKING SUCCESS STRATEGIES

We can't guarantee that students will get higher test scores than they deserve. But if all the right steps are taken, we can nearly guarantee that your students will not perform lower than they should. Learning the content is an obvious step, but make sure you use the suggestions given earlier. First of all, students will need to go through the learning stages that were introduced earlier:

Acquisition

Elaboration

Trial-and-error correction

Meaning making

Memory tools

Rest/settling time

Revision to strengthen memory

Now for the test strategies. Ideally, students would do their final rehearsal under the same testing stress in the same location as the actual test. Students should be given a memory prompt such as a choice of either (a) a peppermint candy to suck on or (b) chewing gum with sugar, not sugar free—the brain needs the glucose. These create a slight smell and taste that can be associated (Barker et al., 2003) with the memories of knowing their material as it is reviewed.

If you associate a particular state with a stimulus (sound, sight, odor, etc.), the two become associated such that one may stimulate the other (LaBar et al., 2001). For test taking, a useful state is confidence, so let's review how it works. There are three stages. First, the initial learning process in class begins. Use no peppermints for that stage. The second stage is the review and rehearsal stage. At this point, students are more confident and should know their material well. Now, pass out the peppermint, and students will suck on it while in a confident state of reviewing what they know. Stage 3 is the actual test taking. Make the peppermint available and allow the peppermint to evoke the positive state from the second stage. But there's more. Give the students a short, brisk walk first, before the actual test. Why? Physical activity produces the brain chemicals that support alertness and working memory (Chaouloff, 1989), both needed for success on tests.

Does this work? Many schools have already used this successfully, and test scores are getting closer to the maximum possible for the ability of the students. Remember, these strategies will not help your student overperform—they can't do better than their actual knowledge. But these strategies help you ensure that the students do not underperform, getting a worse score than they deserve.

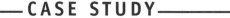

CASE STUDY

Preparing for the Tests

"Our biggest success has been the Pre-SOL (Virginia State Standards of Learning) Test Warm-Up. All classes in the grade level come to the gym at 8:15 a.m. for a half hour of movement before their tests begin. The gym is divided into three stations: a walk/jog track around the outside corner cones and two other aerobic-type activities—one on each half of the gym on the inside of the corner cones.

For three to four minutes, all students are moving to high BPM music. Rotations occur through the three stations on this time frame for 20 minutes. Then all classes sit on the floor and perform their designated stretching, cross-lateral exercises, followed by relaxation. During the last five minutes the students listen to classical music (low BPM). At the end, students are dismissed to their classroom teacher for water breaks before testing begins.

Classroom teachers and administrators are very pleased with the increased attention span the students have while taking the tests. They report the students are better able to focus and stay on task longer. They also report the students are more relaxed and there is less test anxiety. Thanks for everything."

—Mark Pankau, Guilford Elementary School,
Loudoun County Public Schools, Sterling, VA

SYSTEMIC CHANGE: THE NEXT LEVEL

Let's say you've successfully implemented brain-compatible learning into your own curriculum and you would like to see the same success implemented schoolwide or systemwide. Some of the potential challenges you may come up against are the following:

- Other staff may not choose to go in the same direction you have.
- A staff member may have had a bad experience that left a bad taste in his or her mouth.
- A staff member may not grasp the relevancy or is uninspired by the new paradigm.
- Other staff members may fear it will invalidate their past work.
- There is lack of parent, school board, administrative, or community support.
- Staff members may feel that they don't have enough downtime to make the changes.
- There are too many other conflicting priorities and programs.
- There is lack of feedback, or accountability stymies the process.
- There is a lack of sufficient resources, or follow-up impairs process.
- Staff get disheartened due to insufficient acknowledgment and lack of celebration.

BIG-PICTURE ANALYSIS:
TRANSFORMATION HAPPENS

Transformation can occur on many levels: individual, social, cultural, political, and systemwide. Sometimes it even happens without us knowing. Once you transform your own environment and philosophy and are walking the talk on a daily and moment-by-moment basis, others can't help but take notice. Just as the snowball gets bigger rolling downhill, so will the awareness of brain-compatible learning. What works gets embedded.

Though change usually happens gradually, it surely occurs. Though our brain is poorly designed to take on whole new paradigms at once, it is well designed for nibbling away at a concept or building a model over time. Expect systemic change to take time. Meanwhile, you can continue to make gains by

- Identifying your own individual beliefs
- Identifying limiting institutional practices
- Redesigning the purpose, approach, content, and processes in your own curriculum
- Applying your learning; doing your own action research
- Doing big-picture analysis and long-term planning
- Remembering that meaningful transformation takes time

ACTION RESEARCH MAKES A DIFFERENCE!

Action research means applying your knowledge about brain-compatible learning to your own classroom or learning environment. In so doing, remember to keep the following areas in mind:

Instruction

Are your teaching approaches flexible, individualized, based on multiple learning styles, novel, and interesting? Do you ask students to work in teams? Are your assignments fun, realistic, complex, and rich? Do you ensure that students receive lots of feedback on a daily basis?

Curriculum

Is your subject matter relevant, cross-curricular, interdisciplinary, and stage appropriate? Is it examined from many angles over a period of time? Do you present the big picture, as well as the smaller chunks? Is there an emphasis on the process—on learning to learn? Do you include life-skills learning and emotional literacy?

Environment

Is your classroom set up with a variety of seating and temperature options? Do you use music, multiple lighting types, rich visuals, and aromas? Do you have plants in your classroom? If you have classroom pets, are they well cared for? Does your classroom maintain a rule of respect for all individuals and an environment free of threats and tight teacher control?

Assessment

Does your assessment approach take into consideration the uniqueness of the individual learner? Do you assess learning over time, rather than incrementally? Do you include emotional literacy and multiple intelligences in the assessment process? Do you set up structures for peer and personal assessment? Have you eliminated traditional tests, comparisons, and curves? Do you emphasize mental models and give learners some choice in the assessment process?

THE LEARNING COMMUNITY

Schools or "learning communities" that use brain-compatible learning methods outlined in this book are consistently more successful than those that don't. What is meant by successful? There are fewer dropouts, the students enjoy school more, they are willing to take risks, think for themselves, and be creative. They understand how they learn and love to do it. It's more than just applying a few techniques. A school must become a learning organization. In the process of transforming your school into a learning community, consider the following shareholders:

Parents

Have you brought the parents into what you are doing? Do they understand the basic principles of brain-compatible learning? Are they seeing the results of your efforts? Are they being asked to get involved in the classroom as perhaps a guest speaker, volunteer, or contributor? Encourage family support, positive parental feedback, academic involvement, and a home environment that is rich with opportunities for exploration and managed risk.

Teachers

Are you nurturing teachers to support each other? Does every teacher know every other teacher's best ideas? Are you open to their suggestions, feedback, and questions? Are formal and informal structures of support in place? Are you building a collective vision?

Students

Are students included in the decision-making process? Are you providing an environment that is responsive to their goals? Are students allowed to move around freely in the classroom and to work in pairs or groups if they wish? Are students always respected as an important part of the learning organization?

Local Media

Have you notified the various media to elicit stories about your classroom or school? Perhaps you could invite them to an open house or a presentation of special term projects, a schoolwide event, or a guest speaker.

School and District Staff

Find out how others feel about the current state of things. Have you asked your school and district administrators how they think the current system works and how they think teaching and learning works in their area of responsibility? Have you shared your learning with them? Are they familiar with brain-compatible learning strategies? Would they like to learn more? Keep asking why until you find out what investment your organization has in keeping a particular useless policy in place.

A learning organization of the twenty-first century will not necessarily know the best way to do everything; what it will know, however, is how to learn its way into the future. Educators will be committed to the process of making their environments brain compatible, rather than brain antagonistic. Staff members will feel free to speak honestly and to share ideas, there will be respect for differences, teachers will enjoy their profession, and they will delight in their students' success. Does this sound like a place you would like to work? Keep reading!

WHAT'S NEXT?

You're a hungry learner! Now it's time to feed that hunger. Fortunately, we have enough insights to make dramatic and powerful changes in how we conceptualize, plan, and implement educational policy today. While the research doesn't always give us the specific form or structure for how to shift the paradigm, it's clear that we have enough to figure it out ourselves.

Naturally, a book like this is not meant to be the detailed blueprints for change. The discoveries are coming so fast that even the professionals who study this field full time are overwhelmed. But don't wait for more research. The research will just keep coming. It makes more sense to start with what you can do today and take the next step—your own action research. In that process, there are plenty of additional resources for you to refer to along the way.

Good luck as you continue the journey into the brain and how it learns best. And congratulations on completing the first leg of this exciting journey.

APPENDIX A

BRAIN-SMART RESOURCES AND SUPPORT

Brain-Compatible Strategies by Eric Jensen

Get over 500 easy-to-use classroom strategies that purposely engage the brain to boost attention, motivation, learning, meaning, and transfer. Available at corwinpress.com.

Brain-Based Learning by Eric Jensen

The most complete volume on new approaches to discipline, intelligence, memory, attention, learning, and environments. A highly detailed and practical book for all teachers, administrators, and trainers. Fully referenced, easy to use, and well illustrated. Available at corwinpress.com.

How the Brain Learns by David Sousa

This best-selling volume provides more detail on the nitty-gritty, the practical side of applying this knowledge to the classroom. David Sousa is a former teacher and administrator. Available at corwinpress.com.

Brain-Compatible Workshops and Trainings

Eric Jensen conducts workshops and in-depth programs on brain-compatible teaching and learning. These practical development programs are cost efficient, long lasting, and provide in-house resources for your school or district. Call (888) 638-7246 for free information or visit www.jensenlearning.com for training dates and locations.

Learning Brain Expo

See, hear, and experience dozens of the world's top experts linking new brain research with learning, thinking, enrichment, arts, memory, curriculum, physical education, assessment, movement, and music. Highly recommended buffet of choices in an exciting three-day conference! Call (888) 638-7246 for a *free* brochure or log on to www.brainexpo.com for complete conference details.

APPENDIX B

GLOSSARY OF BRAIN TERMINOLOGY

Acetylcholine (uh-see-til-KO-lene) A common memory neurotransmitter, particularly involved in long-term memory formation. Specifically released at key junction points, it's present at higher levels during sleep.

ACTH Also called adrenal-corticotrophin release hormone, this stress-related hormone is produced by the pituitary gland. It's released into our system when we experience injury, emotion, pain, infections, or other trauma.

Adrenaline The hormone of risk, excitement, and urgency. Under stress, fear, or excitement, this hormone is released from our adrenal gland into our bloodstream. When it reaches our liver, it stimulates the release of glucose for rapid energy. Abrupt increases caused by anger can constrict heart vessels, requiring the heart to pump with higher pressure. Also known as epinephrine.

Amygdala (uh-MIG-da-la) Located in the middle of the brain area (anterior temporal lobe), right at the base of the hippocampus. These two almond-shaped structures may be the critical processor area for senses in the same way a smoke detector does in our house. It signals to our brain the emotions of uncertainty, anger, fear, and suspicion. It's connected to the many other areas of the brain and is critical in learning, cognition, and emotional memories.

Astrocytes The largest and most numerous of the supporting, or glial, cells in the brain and spinal cord. Astrocytes (meaning "star cells" because of their shape) help regulate the chemical environment around cells, respond to injury, communicate, and release regulatory substances that influence nerve cells.

Axons The long fibers extending from the brain cells (neurons) that carry the output (an electrical nerve impulse) to other neurons. Can be up to a meter long. When used often enough, axons build up a fatty white insulation called myelin.

Brain stem Located at the top of the spinal cord. Links the lower brain with the middle of the brain and cerebral hemispheres. Often referred to as the lower brain or reptilian brain in MacLean's older (now out of date) triune model.

Broca's area Part of the lower frontal lobe in the cerebrum, right at the border of the temporal lobe. It converts thoughts into sounds (or written words) and sends the message to the motor area to speak.

Cerebellum A cauliflower-shaped structure located below the occipital area and next to the brainstem. The word is Latin for "little brain." Traditionally, research linked it to balance, posture, coordination, sequencing, and muscle movements.

Cerebral cortex The newspaper-sized, ¼"-thick outermost layer of the cerebrum. It's wrinkled, six layers deep, and packed with brain cells (neurons). Cortex is the Latin word for "bark" or "rind." This is the outer covering that we see when we look at the top two-thirds of a brain.

Cerebrum The largest, main assembly of the brain, composed of the left and right hemisphere, and includes the frontal, parietal, temporal, and occipital lobes. It does not include the midbrain areas, the cerebellum, or brain stem.

Cingulate gyrus (SIN-gue-lit GYE-rus) Lies directly between the midbrain areas and the upper forehead. It mediates communication between the cortex and midbrain structures. Involved with right-wrong, decision making. and emotions. It helps us shift from one mind-body state to another.

Corpus callosum A white-matter bundle of 240 million nerve fibers that connect the left and right hemispheres. Located in the top middle of the brain area, below the cortex and above the midbrain area.

Dendrites Similar to our fingers, the strandlike fibers emanating from the cell body. They provide for the input and docking areas for axons when they each connect to make a synapse. Each cell usually has many, many dendrites.

Dopamine A powerful and common neurotransmitter primarily involved in producing positive moods or feelings. It is synthesized from proteins and plays a role in our working memory and movements too. It's commonly in shortage in patients suffering from Parkinson's disease. Remember this by thinking of the word "Yahoo!"

Endorphin A natural opiate. This neurotransmitter is similar to morphine; it is produced in the pituitary gland. Protects against excessive pain and is released with ACTH and enkephalins into the brain. It is released to create the runner's high that dulls the pain of running. It is only released under the perception of pain.

Epinephrine (eh-puh-NEFF-rin) This is also the word for adrenaline (think of the word "Yikes!"). It's a common neurotransmitter, hormone, and neuromodulator primarily involved in our arousal states such as fight, freeze or flight, metabolic rate, blood pressure, emotions, and mood.

Frontal lobes One of four main areas of the cerebrum, the upper, front brain area just above our eyes. Controls voluntary movement, verbal expression, problem solving, will power, judgment, creativity, and planning. As it matures, it inhibits impulsivity and rash actions. The other three areas of the cerebrum are the occipital, parietal, and temporal.

GABA Gamma-aminobutyric acid. This neurotransmitter acts as an inhibitory agent, an off switch. Without this common chemical, neurons would fire indiscrimately, as when we have seizures.

Glia A critically important brain cell. These are one of two types of brain cells (the other is a neuron). These outnumber neurons fivefold to tenfold. They carry nutrients, speed repair, help myelinate, and may form their own communication network. They are also involved in neurogenesis. Short for "neuroglia."

Hippocampus (hip-uh-CAM-pus) Found deep in the temporal lobe. We have two of them, one on each side of the brain. They're highly connected, learn fast, and have small memory. They're crescent-shaped and are strongly involved in learning and memory formation. New learning (explicit) is held here for hours, days, or even weeks before being either discarded or transmitted to the cortex for long-term memory.

Hypothalamus Small structure, right under the thalamus, located in the bottom center of the midbrain area. It serves much like a thermostat. It monitors and regulates appetite, hormone secretion, digestion, sexuality, circulation, emotions, and sleep.

Lateralization Refers to the activity of using much more of one hemisphere than another. The term "relative lateralization" is a bit more accurate, because we are usually using at least some of the left and right hemispheres at the same time.

Limbic system An older term coined by Dr. Paul Maclean in the 1950s. This is a group of connected structures in the midbrain area that include the hypothalamus, amygdala, thalamus, fornix, hippocampus, and cingulate. Not used much; a bit out of date.

Lower brain The lower portion of the brain composed of the upper spinal cord, medulla, pons, and some say the reticular formation. It sorts sensory information and regulates our survival functions like breathing and heart rate.

Medulla Located in the brain stem. It channels information between the cerebral hemispheres and the spinal cord. It controls respiration, circulation, wakefulness, breathing, and heart rate.

Myelin A fatty white shield that coats and insulates axons. It can help make the cells (neurons) more efficient and travel up to 12 times faster. Think of it as the rubber coating on the electrical cords around your house.

Neurogenesis The process of growing new brain cells. In humans it's known to occur only in the hippocampus and olfactory area. It also occurs in birds, rats, monkeys, and humans.

Neuromodulators Chemicals that influence the quality of transmission at the synapse. Examples are cortisol, estrogen, testosterone, or adrenaline. These are the amplifiers of the actual signal (the neurotransmitters).

Neurons One of two types of brain cells—the other is glia. We have about 30 billion to 50 billion neurons and many more glia. Neurons receive stimulation from their branches, known as dendrites. They communicate to other neurons by firing a nerve impulse along an axon.

Neurotransmitters Our brain's biochemical messengers. We have over 50 types of them. These usually act as the stimulus that excites a neighboring neuron or an inhibitor to suppress activation. Examples are serotonin, GABA, and dopamine.

Norepinephrine (nor-EH-pi-neff-rin) A sister hormone of epinephrine (it's the same as noradrenaline). It's a excitatory neuromodulator—primarily involved in our arousal states, triggered by urgency, risk, or excitement (think of the word "Yikes!").

Nucleus basalis (NEW-clee-us bah-SAL-us) Located in the lower midbrain area. This structure is highly implicated in learning and memory. If activated, it seems to tell the rest of the brain that what is being learned is important and to save it. It projects to the amygdala and cortex and triggers acetylcholine release to strengthen memories.

Occipital lobe Located in the rear of the cerebrum. One of the four major areas of the upper brain, this processes our vision. The other three areas are parietal, frontal, and temporal lobes. This is the videocam of our brain—it records the images of life.

Oligodendrocyte (Oh-lig-oh-DEN-dro-cyte) An especially important type of glial cell involved in the support of cells following neurogenesis. It supports myelination.

Oxytocin (Ox-eee-TOE-sin) A peptide also known as the commitment molecule. It's released during sex and pregnancy and influences pair bonding. Females have more than males.

Parietal lobe (puh-RYE-uh-tal lobe) The top of our upper brain. It's one of four major areas of the cerebrum. This area deals with reception of sensory information from the contralateral body side. It also plays a part in reading, writing, language, and calculation. This area is the "circus" area (sensory, spatial, and motor). The other three lobes are the occipital, temporal, and frontal.

Pons Located near the top of the brain stem, above the medulla. It's a critical relay station for our sensory information.

Reticular formation A small structure, located at the top of the brain stem and near the bottom of the middle of the brain. It's the regulator responsible for attention, arousal, and sleep-awake consciousness.

Serotonin A common neurotransmitter, most responsible for inducing relaxation, regulating appetite, mood, learning, consciousness, and sleep (think "ahhhh"). Antidepressants (like Prozac) usually suppress the absorption of serotonin, making it more active.

Synapse The location of the junction area. When an axon of one neuron releases neurotransmitters to stimulate the dendrites of another cell, the resulting junction area of reaction is a synapse. The adult human has trillions! It's the hand-off spot for the electrical to chemical to electrical relay in our brain.

Temporal lobes Located on the side of the cerebrum (in the middle of our upper brain, near our ears). It's an area believed responsible for hearing, senses, language, learning, and memory storage. The other three major cerebrum areas are the frontal, occipital, and parietal lobes. They store words, text, and language. It's the TiVo in our brain.

Thalamus Located deep within the middle of the brain. It's a key sensory relay station for all senses except smell. It's critical to our daily consciousness and memory retrieval. It's the server to our brain.

Vasopressin A stress-related hormone that is synthesized in the hypothalamus. It's correlated with vasoconstriction, blood pressure regulation, water conservation, memory, and distress.

Wernicke's area (WERE-nick-eee's) The upper back edge of the parietal and left temporal lobe. Here the brain converts thoughts into language.

REFERENCES

Abbott, T. (1999) *The hidden stairs and the magic carpet (secrets of Droon).* (T. Jessell, Illus.). New York: Scholastic.

Alexander, J., O'Boyle, M., & Benbow, C. (1966). Developmentally advanced EEG alpha power in gifted male and female adolescents. *International Journal of Psychophysiology, 23*(1–2), 25–31.

Anderson, C. A., & Bushman, B. J. (2001). Effects of violent video games on aggressive behavior, aggressive cognition, aggressive affect, physiological arousal, and prosocial behavior: A meta-analytic review of the scientific literature. *Psychological Science: A Journal of the American Psychological Society, 12*(5), 353–359.

Bailey, C. H., Kandel, E. R., & Si, K. (2004). The persistence of long-term memory: A molecular approach to self-sustaining changes in learning-induced synaptic growth. *Neuron, 44,* 49–57.

Baker, L. A., Vernon, P. A., & Ho, H. Z. (1991). The genetic correlation between intelligence and speed of information processing. *Behavior Genetics, 21*(4), 351–367.

Bardo, M. T. (2004). High-risk behavior during adolescence. *Annals of the New York Academy of Sciences, 1021,* 59–60.

Barker, S., Grayhem, P., Koon, J., Perkins, J., Whalen, A., & Raudenbush, B. (2003). Improved performance on clerical tasks associated with administration of peppermint odor. *Perceptual and Motor Skills, 97*(3 Pt. 1), 1007–1010.

Bellisle, F. (2004). Effects of diet on behavior and cognition in children. *British Journal of Nutrition, 92*(2), S227–S232.

Berezovskii, V. A., Zelenskaia, T. M., Serebrovskaia, T. V., Zverkova, A. S., & Il'chevich, N. V. (1986). Degree of concordance of the adaptive reactions in twins under mountain climate conditions and their relationship to the reactivity of the physiological connective tissue system. *Fiziol Cheloveka, 12*(6), 992–998.

Bogolepova, I. (1994). The cytoarchitectonic characteristics of the speech center of the brain in gifted people in the plan to study individual variability of human brain structure. *Morfologiia, 106*(4–6), 31–38.

Bolger, K., Patterson, D., Thompson, W., & Kupersmidt, J. (1995). Psychosocial adjustment among children experiencing persistent and intermittent family economic hardship. *Child Development, 66,* 1107–1129.

Bower, B. (1987). Memory boost from spaced-out learning. *Science News, 131,* 244.

Bower, B. (1999). The mental butler did it. *Science News, 156,* 280–282

Brown, E., Rush, A., & McEwen, B. (1999). Hippocampal remodeling and damage by corticosteroids: Implications for mood disorders. *Neuropsychopharmacology, 21*, 474–484.

Bunge, S. A., Dudukovic, N. M., Thomason, M. E., Vaidya, C. J., & Gabrieli, J. D. (2002). Immature frontal lobe contributions to cognitive control in children: Evidence from fMRI. *Neuron, 33*(2), 301–311.

Cacioppo, J., Berntson, G., Sheridan, J., & McClintock, M. (2001). Multilevel analyses of human behavior: Social neuroscience and the complementing nature of social and biological approaches. In J. Cacioppo et al. (Eds.), *Foundations of Social Neuroscience* (pp. 21–46). Cambridge: Massachusetts Institute of Technology Press.

Cahill, L., Uncapher, M., Kilpatrick, L., Alkire, M. T., & Turner, J. (2004). Sex-related hemispheric lateralization of amygdala function in emotionally influenced memory: An fMRI investigation. *Learning and Memory, 11*(3), 261–266.

Callicott, J. H., Mattay, V. S., Bertolino, A., Finn, K., Coppola, R., Frank, J. A., et al. (1999). Physiological characteristics of capacity constraints in working memory as revealed by functional MRI. *Cerebral Cortex, 9*(1), 20–26.

Carlson, R., Chandler, P., & Sweller, J. (2003). Learning and understanding science instructional material. *Journal of Educational Psychology, 95*(3), 629–640.

Carraher, T., Carraher, D., & Schliemann, A. (1985). Mathematics in the streets and in the schools. *British Journal of Developmental Psychology, 3*, 21–29.

Carskadon, M. A., Wolfson, A. R., Acebo, C., Tzischinsky, O., & Seifer, R. (1998). Adolescent sleep patterns, circadian timing, and sleepiness at a transition to early school days. *Sleep, 21*(8), 871–881.

Carter, H. (1999). Couch potato culture starts in the cradle. *Newswise.* Retrieved November 4, 2005, from www.dialogueworks.co.uk/newswise/months/apri199/cojun.html

Castellanos, F., & Acosta, M. (2002). The neuroanatomy of attention deficit/hyperactivity disorder. *Revista de neurologia, 38*(1), S131–S136.

Ceci, S. J., & Roazzi, A. (1994). The effects of context on cognition: Postcards from Brazil. In R. J. Sternberg & R. K. Wagner (Eds.), *Mind in context: Interactionist perspectives on human intelligence* (pp. 74–101). New York: Cambridge University Press.

Champagne, F. A., & Curley, J. P. (2005). How social experiences influence the brain. *Current Opinion in Neurobiology, 15*(6), 704–709.

Chaouloff, F. (1989). Physical exercise and brain monoamines: A review. *Acta Physiologica Scandinavica, 137*, 1–13.

Chi, M. T. H., Feltovich, P., & Glaser, R. (1981). Categorization and representation of physics problems by experts and novices. *Cognitive Science, 5*, 121–152.

Christakis, D. A., Zimmerman, F. J., DiGiuseppe, D. L., & McCarty, C. A. (2004). Early television exposure and subsequent attentional problems in children. *Pediatrics, 113*(4), 708–713.

Chugani, H. (1998). A critical period of brain development: Studies of cerebral glucose utilization with PET. *Preventive Medicine, 27*(2), 184–188.

Coffey, C. E., Lucke, J. F., Saxton, J. A., Ratcliff, G., Unitas, L. J., Billig, B., et al. (1998). Sex differences in brain aging: A quantitative magnetic resonance imaging study. *Archives of Neurology, 55*, 169–179.

Colicos, M. A., Collins, B. E., Sailor, M. J., & Goda, Y. (2001). Remodeling of synaptic actin induced by photoconductive stimulation. *Cell, 107*(5), 605-616.

Collins, D. W., & Kimura, D. (1997). A large sex difference on a two-dimensional mental rotation task. *Behavioral Neuroscience, 111*, 845–849.

Cowan, N. (2001). The magical number 4 in short-term memory: A reconsideration of mental storage capacity. *Behavioral and Brain Sciences, 24*(1), 87–114.

Damasio, A. (1994). *Descartes' error.* New York: Grosset/Putnam.

Davatzikos, C., & Resnick, S. M. (1998). Sex differences in anatomic measures of interhemispheric connectivity: Correlations with cognition in women, but not men. *Cerebral Cortex, 8*, 635–640.

Delgado, A. R., & Prieto, G. (1996). Sex differences in visuospatial ability: Do performance factors play such an important role? *Memory and Cognition, 24*, 504–510.

Denenberg, V. H., Kim, D. S., & Palmiter, R. D. (2004). The role of dopamine in learning, memory, and performance of a water escape task. *Behavioral Brain Research, 148*(1–2), 73–78.

Diamond, D., Park, C., Hemen, K., & Rose, G. (1999). Exposing rats to a predator impairs spatial working memory in the radial arm water maze. *Hippocampus, 9*, 542–552.

Di Vesta, F. J., & Smith, D. A. (1979). The pausing principle: Increasing the efficiency of memory for ongoing events. *Contemporary Educational Psychology, 4*(3), 288–296.

Dolcos, F., & McCarthy, G. (2006). Brain systems mediating cognitive interference by emotional distraction. *Journal of Neuroscience, 26*(7), 2072–2079.

Draganski, B., Gaser, C., Kempermann, G., Kuhn, H. G., Winkler, J., Büchel, C., et al. (2006). Temporal and spatial dynamics of brain structure changes during extensive learning. *Journal of Neuroscience, 26*(23), 6314–6317.

Dudai, Y. (2004). The neurobiology of consolidations, or, how stable is the engram? *Annual Review of Psychology, 55*, 51–86.

Durston, S., Hulshoff-Pol, H. E., & Casey, B. J. (2001). Anatomical MRI of the developing human brain: What have we learned? *Journal of the American Academy of Child and Adolescent Psychiatry, 40*, 1012–1020.

Eldridge, B., Galea, M., McCoy, A., Wolfe, R., & Graham, H. K. (2003). Uptime normative values in children aged 8 to 15 years. *Developmental Medicine & Child Neurology, 45*(3), 189–193.

Epel, E., Blackburn, E., Lin, J., Dhabhar, F., Adler, N., Morrow, J., et al. (2004). Accelerated telomere shortening in response to life stress. *Proceedings of the National Academy of Sciences of the United States of America, 101*(49), 17312–17315.

Ericsson, K. A. (1996). The acquisition of expert performance. In K. A. Ericsson (Ed.), *The road to excellence: The acquisition of expert performance in the arts, science and games.* Mahwah, NJ: Lawrence Erlbaum.

Eriksson, P. S., Perfilieva, E., Bjork-Eriksson, T., Alborn, A. M., Nordborg, C., Peterson, D. A., et al. (1998). Neurogenesis in the adult human hippocampus. *Nature Medicine, 4*(11), 1313–1317.

Farber, N. B., & Olney, J. W. (2003). Drugs of abuse that cause developing neurons to commit suicide. *Developmental Brain Research, 147*(1–2), 37–45.

Fields, J. M., & Casper, L. M. (2001). America's families and living arrangements: March 2000. In *U.S. Census Bureau Current Population Reports P20–537.* Washington, DC: U.S. Government Printing Office.

Fiske, E. (Ed.). (1999). Champions of change: The impact of arts on learning. *The Arts Education Partnership.* Retrieved February 22, 2006, from www .artsedge.kennedy-center.org/champions

Fox, M., Pac, S., Devaney, B., & Jankowski, L. (2004). Feeding infants and toddlers study: What foods are infants and toddlers eating? *Journal of the American Dietetic Association, 104*(1), 22–30.

Fox, N. A., Henderson, H. A., Marshall, P. J., Nichols, K. E., & Ghera, M. M. (2005). Behavioral inhibition: Linking biology and behavior within a developmental framework. *Annual Review of Psychology, 56,* 235–262.

Frank, D. A., & Greenberg, M. E. (1994). CREB: A mediator of long-term memory from mollusks to mammals. *Cell, 79,* 5–8.

Frank, L., Stanley, G., & Brown, E. (2004). Hippocampal plasticity across multiple days of exposure to novel environments. *Journal of Neuroscience, 24*(35), 7681–7689.

Furrer, C., & Skinner, E. (2003). Sense of relatedness as a factor in children's academic engagement and performance. *Journal of Educational Psychology, 95*(1), 148–162.

Fuster, J. (1995). *Memory in the cerebral cortex.* Cambridge: Massachusetts Institute of Technology Press.

Gaser, C., & Schlaug, G. (2003). Brain structures differ between musicians and non-musicians. *Journal of Neuroscience, 23,* 9240–9245.

Gazzaniga, M. (1988). *Mind matters: How mind and brain interact to create our conscious lives.* Boston: Houghton-Mifflin/Massachusetts Institute of Technology Press.

Goda, Y., & Davis, G. W. (2003). Mechanisms of synapse assembly and disassembly. *Neuron, 40*(2), 243–264.

Goodman, J. S., Wood, R. E., & Hendrickx, M. (2004). Feedback specificity, exploration, and learning. *Journal of Applied Psychology, 89*(2), 248–262.

Gordon, H. W., Stoffer, D. S., & Lee, P. A. (1995). Ultradian rhythms in performance on tests of specialized cognitive function. *International Journal of Neuroscience, 83*(3–4), 199–211.

Gould, E., McEwen, B., Tanapat, P., Galea, L., & Fuchs, E. (1997). Neurogenesis in the dentate gyrus of the adult tree shrew is regulated by psychosocial stress and NMDA receptor activation. *Journal of Neuroscience, 17,* 2492–2498.

Guay, F., Boivin, M., & Hodges, E. (1999). Predicting change in academic achievement: A model of peer experiences and self-system processes. *Journal of Educational Psychology, 91*(1), 105–115.

Gunnar, M. (2000). Early adversity and the development of stress reactivity and regulation. In C. Nelson & N. Mahwah (Eds.), *The effects of adversity on neurobehavioral development: Minnesota symposia on child psychology* (Vol. 31, pp. 163–200). Minneapolis, MN: Lawrence Erlbaum.

Haier, R. J., Siegel, B. V. Jr, MacLachlan, A., Soderling, E., Lottenberg, S., & Buchsbaum, M. S. (1992). Regional glucose metabolic changes after learning a complex visuospatial/motor task: A positron emission tomographic study. *Brain Research, 570*(1–2), 134–143.

Harasty, J., Double, K. L., Halliday, G. M., Kril, J. J., & McRitchie, D. A. (1997). Language-associated cortical regions are proportionally larger in the female brain. *Archives of Neurology, 54*, 171–176.

Heilman, K. (2000). Emotional experience: A neurological model. In R. Lane & L. Nadel (Eds.), *The cognitive neuroscience of emotion* (pp. 328–344). New York: Oxford University Press.

Heschong Mahone Group. (2003). *Windows and classrooms: A study of student performance and the indoor environment.* Retrieved September 2, 2006, from www.h-m-g.com/daylighting/main.htm

Hirsch-Pasek, K., Eyer, D., & Golinkoff, R. M. (2003). *Einstein never used flash cards: How our children really learn—And why they need to play more and memorize less.* Emmaus, PA: Rodale Press.

Hoffman, A. (1996). *Schools, violence, and society.* Westport, CT: Praeger.

Hopf, F., Waters, J., Mehta, S., & Smith, S. (2002). Stability and plasticity of developing synapses in hippocampal neuronal cultures. *Journal of Neuroscience, 22*(3), 775–781.

House, J., Landis, K., & Umberson, D. (1988). Social relationships and health. *Science, 241*, 540–545.

Hu, P., & Young, J. (1999). *Summary of travel trends: 1995 nationwide personal transportation survey.* Retrieved November 2, 2005, from www.cta.ornl.gov/npts/1995/Doc/trends_report.pdf

Huttenlocher, J., Levine, S., & Vevea, J. (1998). Environmental input and cognitive growth: A study using time-period comparisons. *Child Development, 69*(4), 1012–1029.

Jacobs, B., Schall, M., & Scheibel, A. (1993). A quantitative dendritic analysis of Bernice's area in humans II: Gender, hemispheric and environmental factor. *Journal of Comparative Neurology, 327*, 97–111.

Jausovec, N., & Jausovec, K. (2004). Differences in induced brain activity during the performance of learning and working-memory tasks related to intelligence. *Brain and Cognition, 54*(1), 65–74.

Jensen, E. (2000). *Different brains, different learners.* Thousand Oaks, CA: Corwin Press.

Jensen, E. (2006). *Enriching the brain.* San Francisco: Jossey-Bass/Wiley.

Johnson, J., Cohen, P., Smailes, E., Kasen, S., & Brook, J. (2002). Television viewing and aggressive behavior during adolescence and adulthood. *Science, 295*(5564), 2468–2471.

Johnson-Laird, P. N. (1980). Mental models in cognitive science. *Cognitive Science, 4*, 71–115.

Joy, L. A., Kimball, M., & Zabrack, M. L. (1986). Television exposure and children's aggressive behavior. In T. M. Williams (Ed.), *The impact of television: A natural experiment involving three towns* (pp. 303–360). New York: Academic Press.

Kennedy, D. O., & Scholey, A. B. (2000). Glucose administration, heart rate and cognitive performance: Effects of increasing mental effort. *Psychopharmacology, 149*(1), 63–71.

Kilberg, M. S., Pan, Y. X., Chen, H., & Leung-Pineda, V. (2005). Nutritional control of gene expression: How mammalian cells respond to amino acid limitation. *Annual Review of Nutrition, 25*, 59–85.

Kilgard, M., & Merzenich, M. (1998). Cortical map reorganization enabled by nucleus basalis activity. *Science, 279*, 1714–1718.

Killgore, W. D., Oki, M., & Yurgelun-Todd, D. A. (2001). Sex-specific developmental changes in amygdala responses to affective faces. *Neuroreport, 12*(2), 427–433.

Kluger, A., & DeNisi, A. (1996). The effects of feedback interventions on performance: A historical review, a meta-analysis, and a preliminary feedback intervention theory. *Psychological Bulletin, 119*(2), 254–284.

Koenen, K., Moffitt, T., Caspi, A., Taylor, A., & Purcell, S. (2003). Domestic violence is associated with environmental suppression of IQ in young children. *Development and Psychopathology, 15*(2), 297–311.

LaBar, K. S., Gitelman, D. R., Parrish, T. B., Kim, Y. H., Nobre, A. C., & Mesulam, M. M. (2001). Hunger selectively modulates corticolimbic activation to food stimuli in humans. *Behavioral Neuroscience, 115*(2), 493–500.

Lane, R., & Nadel, L. (Eds.). (2000). *The cognitive neuroscience of emotion.* New York: Oxford University Press.

Larson, R. W., & Verma, S. (1999). How children and adolescents spend time across the world: Work, play, and developmental opportunities. *Psychological Bulletin, 125*(6), 701–736.

Latham, A. S. (1997). Learning through feedback. *Educational Leadership, 54*(8), 86–87.

Levin, J. R. (1988). Elaboration-based learning strategies: Powerful theory = powerful application. *Contemporary Educational Psychology, 13*(3), 191–205.

Lewit, E. M., Terman, D. L., & Behrman, R. E. (1997). Children and poverty: Analysis and recommendations. *The Future of Children, 7*, 4–24.

Lino, M., Basiotis, P. P., Gerrior, S. A., & Carlson, A. (2002). The quality of young children's diets. *Family Economics and Nutrition Review, 14*(1), 52–60.

Maguire, E. A., Spiers, H. J., Good, C. D., Hartley, T., Frackowiak, R. S., & Burgess, N. (2003). Navigation expertise and the human hippocampus: A structural brain imaging analysis. *Hippocampus, 13*(2), 250–259.

Mahoney, J., Lord, H., & Carryl, E. (2005). An ecological analysis of after-school program participation and the development of academic performance and motivational attributes for disadvantaged children. *Child Development, 76*(4), 811–825.

Maquet, P., Peigneux, P., Laureys, S., & Smith, C. (2002). Be caught napping: You're doing more than resting your eyes. *Nature Neuroscience, 5*(7), 618–619.

Maughan, R. J. (2003). Impact of mild dehydration on wellness and on exercise performance. *European Journal of Clinical Nutrition, 57*(2), S19–S23.

McNamara, D. S. (2001). Reading both high-coherence and low-coherence texts: Effects of text sequence and prior knowledge. *Canadian Journal of Experimental Psychology, 55*(1), 51–62.

Meaney, M., Sapolsky, R., & McEwen, B. (1985). The development of the glucocorticoid receptor system in the rat limbic brain II: An autoradiographic study. *Developmental Brain Research, 18*, 159–164.

Mednick, S. C., Nakayama, K., Cantero, J. L., Atienza, M., Levin, A. A., Pathak, N., et al. (2002). The restorative effect of naps on perceptual deterioration. *Nature Neuroscience, 5*(7), 677–681.

Mednick, S., Nakayama, K., & Stickgold, R. (2003). Sleep-dependent learning: A nap is as good as a night. *Nature Neuroscience, 6*(7), 697–698.

Miczek, K. A., Fish, E. W., De Bold, J. F., & De Almeida, R. M. (2002) Social and neural determinants of aggressive behavior: Pharmacotherapeutic targets at serotonin, dopamine and gamma-aminobutyric acid systems. *Psychopharmacology 163*(3–4), 434–458.

Mogg, K., Bradley, B., & Hallowell, N. (1994). Attentional bias to threat: Roles of trait anxiety, stressful events, and awareness. *Quarterly Journal of Experimental Psychology. Section A, Human Experimental Psychology, 47*(4), 841–864.

Moore, G., & Lackney, J. (1993). School design. *Children's Environments, 10,* 99–112.

Murray, J. (1994). The impact of televised violence. *Hofstra Law Review, 22,* 809–825.

National Center on Addiction and Substance Abuse at Columbia University. (2005). *Under the counter: The diversion and abuse of controlled prescription drugs in the U.S.* New York: Author.

Nettles, S., Mucherah, W., & Jones, D. (2000). Understanding resiliencies: The role of social resources. *Journal of Education for Students Placed at Risk, 5*(1, 2), 47–60.

Padgett, D. A., & Glaser, R. (2003). How stress influences the immune response. *Trends in Immunology, 24*(8), 444–448.

Paus, T., Zijdenbos, A., Worsley, K., Collins, D. L., Blumenthal, J., Geidd, J. N., et al. (1999). Structural maturation of neural pathways in children and adolescents: In vivo study. *Science, 283,* 1908–1911.

Pert, C. B. (1998). *Molecules of emotion.* New York: Simon & Schuster.

Pollitt, E., Gorman, K., Engle, P., Rivera, J., & Martorelli, R. (1995). Nutrition in early life and the fulfillment of intellectual potential. *Journal of Nutrition, 125,* S1111–S1118.

Pomerantz, E. M., Altermatt, E. R., & Saxon, J. L. (2002). Making the grade but feeling distressed: Gender differences in academic performance and internal distress. *Journal of Educational Psychology, 94*(2), 396–404.

Raine, A., Reynolds, C., Venables, P., & Mednick, S. (2002). Stimulation seeking and intelligence: A prospective longitudinal study. *Journal of Personality & Social Psychology, 82*(4), 663–674.

Ramey, S. L., & Ramey, C. T. (2000). Early childhood experiences and developmental competence. In J. Waldfogel & S. Danziger (Eds.), *Securing the future: Investing in children from birth to college* (pp. 122–150). New York: Russell Sage Foundation.

Rauscher, F. H., Shaw, G. L., Levine, L. J., Ky, K. N., & Wright, E. L. (1993). Music and spatial task performance. *Nature, 365,* 611.

Rideout, V., & Vandewater, E. (2003). *Zero to six: Electronic media in the lives of infants and toddlers and preschoolers.* Retrieved August 28, 2006, from www .kff.org/entmedia/ entmedia102803nr.cfm

Rossi, E. (2002). *The psychobiology of gene expression.* New York: W. W. Norton.

Schacter, D. (2001). *The seven sins of memory.* Boston: Houghton-Mifflin.

Schlaepfer, T. E., Harris, G. J., Tien, A. Y., Peng, L., Lee, S., & Pearlson, G. D. (1995). Structural differences in the cerebral cortex of healthy female and male subjects: A magnetic resonance imaging study. *Psychiatry Research, 61,* 129–135.

Schneider, M. (2002). *Do school facilities affect academic outcomes?* Washington, DC: National Clearing House for Educational Facilities.

Schore, A. N. (2000). Attachment and the regulation of the right brain. *Attachment and Human Development, 2*(1), 23–47.

Schroth, M. L. (1997). Effects of frequency of feedback on transfer in concept identification. *American Journal of Psychology, 110*(1), 71–79.

Shadmehr, R., & Holcomb, H. H. (1997). Neural correlates of motor memory consolidation. *Science, 277*(5327), 821–825.

Shannon, B. J., & Buckner, R. L. (2004). Functional-anatomic correlates of memory retrieval that suggest nontraditional processing roles for multiple distinct regions within posterior parietal cortex. *Journal of Neuroscience, 24,* 10084–10092

Simpson, J. Jr., Snyder, A., Gusnard, D., & Raichle, M. (2001). Emotion-induced changes in human medial prefrontal cortex: I. During cognitive task performance. *Proceedings of the National Academy of Sciences, 98*(2), 683–687.

Sowell, E. R., Trauner, D. A., Gamst, A., & Jernigan, T. L. (2002). Development of cortical and subcortical brain structures in childhood and adolescence: A structural MRI study. *Developmental Medicine and Child Neurology, 44*(1), 4–16.

Stahl, R. J. (1994). Using "think-time" and "wait-time" skillfully in the classroom. Tempe: Arizona State University (ERIC Digest ED370885). Retrieved January 1, 2007, from www.ed.gov/databases/ERIC Digests/ed370885.html

Steinberg, L. (2005). Cognitive and affective development in adolescence. *Trends in Cognitive Science, 9*(2), 69–74.

Strasburger, V. C., & Donnerstein, E. (2000). Children, adolescents, and the media in the 21st century. *Adolescent Medicine, 11*(1), 51–68.

Tanaka, S. (2002). Dopamine controls fundamental cognitive operations of multi-target spatial working memory. *Neural Networks, 15*(4–6), 573–582.

Tansey, M. A., Tansey, J. A., & Tachiki, K. H. (1994). Electroencephalographic cartography of conscious states. *International Journal of Neuroscience, 77*(1–2), 89–98.

Thompson, P. M., Giedd, J. N., Woods, R. P., MacDonald, D., Evans, A. C., & Toga, A. W. (2000). Growth patterns in the developing brain detected by using continuum mechanical tensor maps. *Nature, 404*(6774), 190–193.

Uchino, B., Cacioppo, J., & Kiecolt-Glaser, J. (1996). The relationship between social support and physiological process: A review with emphasis on underlying mechanisms and implications for health. *Psychological Bulletin, 119,* 488–531.

U.S. Census Bureau. (1998). Unpublished tables. In *Marital status and living arrangements: March 1998 (Update) P20–514.* Washington, DC: Author. Retrieved December 2002, from www.census.gov/prod/99pubs/p20-514u.pdf

U.S. Department of Transportation, Bureau of Transportation Statistics. (2006). *National household travel survey, 2001–2002.* Retrieved January 1, 2007, from www.bts.gov/publications/the_changing_face_of_transportation and http://www.bts.gov/programs/national_household_travel_survey/daily_travel.html

Wesseling, J. F., & Lo, D. C. (2002). Limit on the role of activity in controlling the release-ready supply of synaptic vesicles. *Journal of Neuroscience, 22*(22), 9708–9720.

Wessler, S. (2004). It's hard to learn when you're scared. *Educational Leadership, 61*(1), 40–43.

Wildey, M. B., Pampalone, S. Z., Pettetier, R. L., Zive, M. M., Elder, J. P., & Sallis, J. F. (2000). Fat and sugar levels are high in snacks purchased from student stores in middle schools. *Journal of the American Dietetic Association, 100*(3), 319–322.

Willoughby, T., Porter, L., Belsito, L., & Yearsley, T. (1999). Use of elaboration strategies by students in grades two, four, and six. *Elementary School Journal, 99*(3), 221–231.

Wiltgen, B. J., Brown, R. A., Talton, L. E., & Silva, A. J. (2004). New circuits for old memories; The role of the neocortex in consolidation. *Neuron, 44*(1), 101–108.

Witelson, S. F., Glezer, I. I., & Kigar, D. L. (1995). Women have greater density of neurons in posterior temporal cortex. *Journal of Neuroscience, 15*, 3418–3428.

INDEX

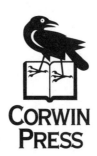

CORWIN PRESS

The Corwin Press logo—a raven striding across an open book—represents the union of courage and learning. Corwin Press is committed to improving education for all learners by publishing books and other professional development resources for those serving the field of PreK–12 education. By providing practical, hands-on materials, Corwin Press continues to carry out the promise of its motto: **"Helping Educators Do Their Work Better."**